# DIVING and SNOR
# the Sea of Cortez

## The Most Complete Guide to Baja California's Best Sites - Includes the Islas de Revillagigedo (Socorro Islands)

Susan Speck and Bruce Williams

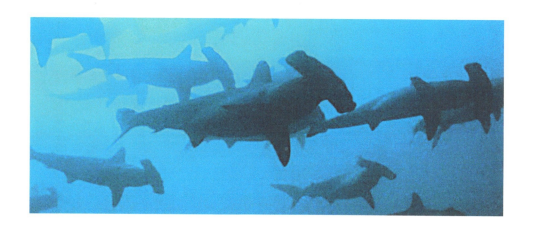

*AuthorHouse™*
*1663 Liberty Drive, Suite 200*
*Bloomington, IN 47403*
*www.authorhouse.com*
*Phone: 1-800-839-8640*

*AuthorHouse™ UK Ltd.*
*500 Avebury Boulevard*
*Central Milton Keynes, MK9 2BE*
*www.authorhouse.co.uk*
*Phone: 08001974150*

This Book Can Be Ordered Directly from Authorhouse
Ph: 888-280-7715      Fax: 812-961-3134
bkorders@authorhouse.com

*First published by AuthorHouse 4/16/2007*

*ISBN: 978-1-4259-3202-2 (sc)*

Please Note: The authors have tried to make the information as accurate as possible. The reader should bear in mind that dive site terrain and landmarks can change over time.  They accept No responsibility for any loss, injury or inconvenience sustained by any person using this book for reference.

*Printed in the United States of America*
*Bloomington, Indiana*

*This book is printed on acid-free paper.*

*Cover: A red shrimp forages on the reef at night.  'by Susan Speck'*
*Title page: Hammerhead sharks*

*All photographs are by the authors.*

Bloomington, IN  Milton Keynes, UK

authorHOUSE®

*This Book Can Be Ordered Directly from Authorhouse*
*Ph: 888-519-5121      Fax: 812-961-1023*

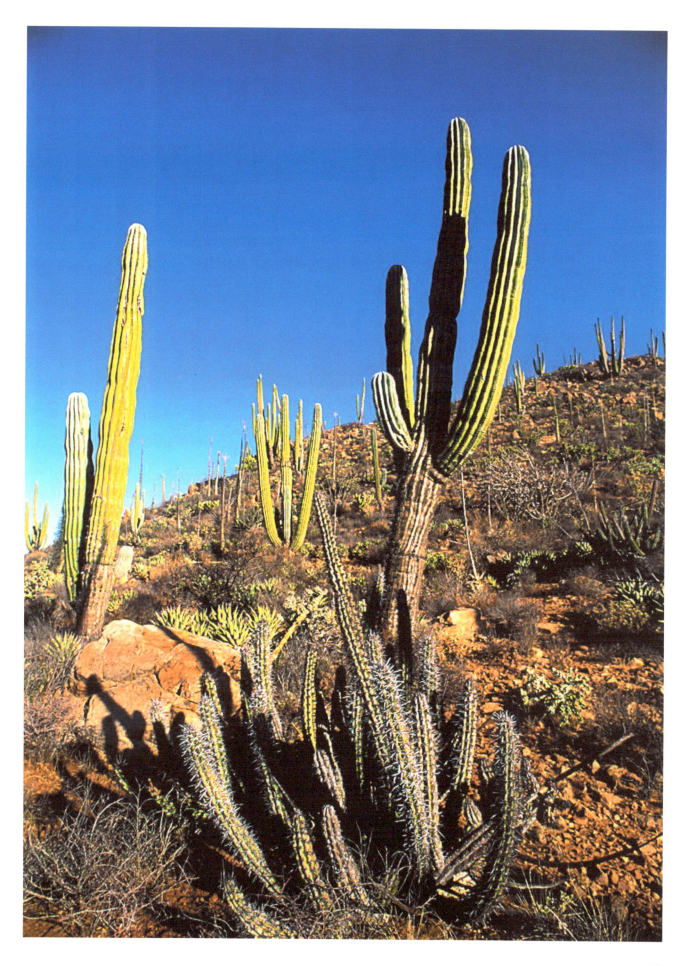

# CONTENTS

# CHAPTER VII

## LORETO

*About the Area*
*Getting There*
*Accommodations*
*Camping*
*Launch Ramps*
*Diving Facilities*
*Diving and Snorkeling*
*Map*

### Dive Sites

23.  *Isla Coronado*
     *23A. Piedra Blanca – 23B. Las*
     *Lagrimas – 23C. La Lobera*
24.  *Isla Carmen*
     *24A. La Cholla – 24B. Punta*
     *Lobos – 24C. Punta Tintorera*
     *24D. Los Picachos*
     *24E. Punta Baja*
     *24F. Punta Colorado*
     *24G. Tuna Boat Wreck*
25.  *Isla Danzante*
     *25A. Faro Norte*
     *25B. Piedra Partida*
     *25C. Piedra Submarino*
     *25D. Los Candeleros*
26.  *Isla Monserrate*
27.  *Isla Catalina*
     *27A. East Side*
     *27B. West Side*
28.  *Punta Coyote*
29.  *Mine Sweeper Wreck*

# CHAPTER VIII

## LA PAZ

*About the Area*
*Getting There*
*Accommodations*
*Camping*
*Launch Ramps*
*Diving Facilities*
*Diving and Snorkeling*
*Map*

### Dive Sites

30.  *Isla Espiritu Santo and*
     *Isla Partida*
     *30A. Punta Lobos*
31.  *Isla Los Islotes*
32.  *El Bajo Seamounts*
33.  *Isla Las Animas*
     *33A. The Island*
34.  *The Pinnacles*
35.  *The Seamount*
36.  *Isla San Diego*
37.  *Salvatierra Wreck*
38.  *La Paz Shoreline*

# CHAPTER IX

## EAST CAPE

*About the Area*
*Getting There*
*Accommodations*
*Camping*
*Launch Ramps*
*Diving Facilities*
*Diving and Snorkeling*
*Map*

### Dive Sites

39.  *Punta Pescadero*
40.  *Cabo Pulmo Reef*
41.  *Colima Wreck*
42.  *El Bajo*
43.  *Los Frailes Bay and*
     *Submarine Canyon*
44.  *Gorda Bank*

# CHAPTER X

## CABO SAN LUCAS

*About the Area*
*Getting There*
*Accommodations*
*Camping*
*Launch Ramps*
*Diving Facilities*
*Diving and Snorkeling*
*Map*

### Dive Sites

45.  *Anegada Rock and*
     *the Sandfalls*
46.  *Land's End*
47.  *The Blowhole*
48.  *The Pinnacle and Rookery*
49.  *Lover's Cove*
50.  *Santa Maria Cove*
51.  *Shipwreck Beach*
52.  *Chileno Beach*

# CHAPTER XI

## SOCORRO ISLANDS

*(Isla de Revillagigedo)*
*About the Area*
*Getting There*
*Diving and Snorkeling*
*Map*

### Dive Sites

53.  *Isla San Benedicto  Boilers*
54.  *Isla San Benedicto  South End*
55.  *Isla Socorro  North End*
56.  *Isla Socorro  O'Neal Rock*
57.  *Isla Socorro  Double Pinnacle*
58.  *Isla Roca Partida*

## APPENDIX

*SCUBA DIVING CENTERS*

## INDEX

### Dedication and Memory of 'Orca-anne'

This book is dedicated and in memory of our 16 ½ yr. old 6lb yorkshire terrier named (Orca). She was a dive club mascot in Calif. for many years and even received a certificate as a 'Colorado River Diver'! She couldn't wait for the boat to stop so she could belly-flop off the stern, riding on snorkelers backs and swimming until she exhaustedly & reluctantly had to climb back on the boat from her specially made teak swimstep. Orca spent many years on the Sea of Cortez. Boating, swimming & exploring were what she lived for. Always living up to her name as a fearless little trooper, she is greatly missed with her passing in July 2005. But her memory will live on in ours and many others hearts forever…

"we love you Orc… thank you "

# FOREWORD

*The great world dropped away very quickly. We lost the fear and fierceness and contagion of war and economic uncertainty. The matters of great importance we had left were not important. There must be an infective quality in these things. We had lost the virus, or it had been eaten by the anti-bodies of quiet.* __

*John Steinbeck, The Log From The Sea of Cortez*

This parched, rugged and primitive peninsula stretches a thousand miles and consists of mountain landscapes with pine trees, immense valleys of cactus forests and vast areas of volcanic craters. Here you can experience sleeping under the eerie moonlit shadows of a 300 yr. old 60ft high (18m) cardon cactus, while your ears fill with the echoing sounds of wailing coyotes in the distance. And in springtime when bursts of rain showers stop suddenly and huge rainbows appear you can see the desert come alive with the pastel colors of wildflowers and thousands of monarch butterflies. It's nature at its best.

On Baja's eastern shore the great Sea of Cortez serpentines the coastline; where empty sandy shoreline is broken up by small towns and fishing camps. Offshore, uninhabited islands jut up from the sea.

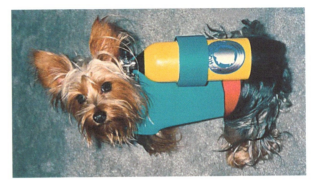

They host many species of animals and serve as nesting grounds for thousands of sea birds. Several species of whales and dolphins live throughout this amazing body of water. Marine life is prolific with its submerged seamounts, walls, caves and reefs.

We have driven the length of Baja California, flown low above much of its coastline in small planes, lived on its water for weeks at a time, and camped along its shorelines. In this book, we have shared with you many of the Sea of Cortez's best known dive sites as well as some that are remote and rarely visited.

Through the years, we have witnessed the great toll that unregulated fishing and the use of gill nets and purse dredges have taken on the Sea of Cortez. Today, the local people are beginning to recognize what their greatest asset is and underwater parks are beginning to be formed. This great body of water is an incredible and fragile ecosystem which needs to be nurtured, for when one part begins to vanish it is only a matter of time before the rest follows. No matter how many times we dive the Sea of Cortez, our fascination is renewed, and like John Steinbeck,… our worldly cares disappear.

Susan Speck
Loreto, B.C.S. April, 2006

A Baja Reality Reminder……'Imagination is more important than information' (Albert Einstein)

# Chapter I   ABOUT BAJA CALIFORNIA

*A Baja reality reminder... 'Life is a journey, not a destination'*

## HISTORY

Baja California is by far one of Mexico's last frontiers. Emerging from its past of over twenty millions years ago, this great peninsula has gone through major geological changes. Massive uplifting and collapses of the ocean floor gradually separated a land mass from Mexico's mainland. Presently, the Baja peninsula continues northwestward, the sea cutting and growing in length. The San Andreas Fault is to be thanked for this relatively new sea. Swinging several inches out per year, *someday we may be able to even drive halfway to Hawaii*! Going through the ice age and then meltdowns, the Sea of Cortez is now at the highest level it has ever been.

Once a scene of steamy erupting volcanoes and torrential downpours, it was a land of palm jungles, ferns, lush vegetation and some species of dinosaur. Camels and mastodons roamed freely as did the 50ft (15m) 23-ton duckbill hadrosaur.

The earliest evidence of human habitation is of the San Dieguito Indians dating back to over 9000 years ago. Early tools and cave paintings have documented their presence. In pre-Hispanic times, nomadic Indian tribes lived along the Pacific coast of Baja, living off the land by fishing and clamming. Even today, Indians come annually from Mexico's mainland to continue an age old heritage of clamming.

In 1535, the Spanish arrived under Hernan Cortez after reports of fabulous pearls to be found. They tried to form a colony near La Paz but were eventually driven out due to lack of supplies and hostile natives. In 1697, the first California mission, Nuestra Senora de Loreto, was founded in Loreto. This was the start of the Jesuit missionary period which lasted until 1767 and produced twenty missions. From 1774 to 1834 eight more missions were built by the Dominican Order. Spanish land grants were given in the early 1800's and small farms and ranches were started. Sadly, by mid-century, the native Indian population had been decimated by European diseases and the Baja missions were abandoned for points north.

The Mexican-American war ended in 1848 with a treaty that divided California between the two countries. Later at the turn of the century, a big boom of gold, silver, copper and gypsum hit and Santa Rosalita became the largest copper mining and smelting operation in Mexico.

Northern Baja became Mexico's 29th state, Baja California Norte in 1952 after it reached the 80,000 population mark needed for statehood. Before 1973, when Highway 1, the Transpeninsular Highway was completed, only rugged dirt roads could get you to your next destination. Driving from Tijuana to La Paz took about two weeks. The now paved highway has contributed to the modernization of this great frontier. Southern Baja reached its 80,000 population mark in less than a year after the highway was completed, which then turned this southern territory into Mexico's 30th state, Baja California Sur.

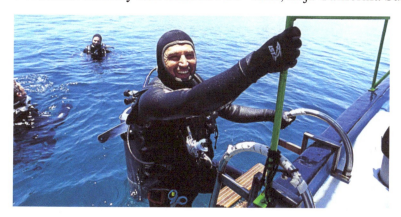

1

## BAJA TODAY

Today, Highway 1 winds serpentinely for 1,000 miles (1,613 km) from the U.S. border to the tip of Cabo San Lucas. It skirts by the cool waters of the Pacific Ocean on its western side; other stretches cross arroyos, up mountains to an elevation of 3200 ft. (970m) before dropping back into desert jungles. With a fascinating array of desert life, many of the plant species are endemic only to this area. The mid-section overlooks the warm waters of the Sea of Cortez, eventually sweeping back to the center, then south to La Paz and beyond. It swings southeast again past the Tropic of Cancer to Cabo San Lucas (Land's End), where the Pacific merges with the Sea of Cortez.

The population of all of Baja is approximately 2.85 million, of which over 85% lives above the 28th parallel in Baja California Norte. Between the major towns, small villages dot the peninsula. Fishing, tourism and farming are Baja's main source of revenue. Most tourism is concentrated in Tijuana and Ensenada in the north and Mulege, Loreto, La Paz, East Cape and Cabo San Lucas in the south. For the most part, much of Baja has been little spoiled by the hand of man which is what makes it so wonderful.

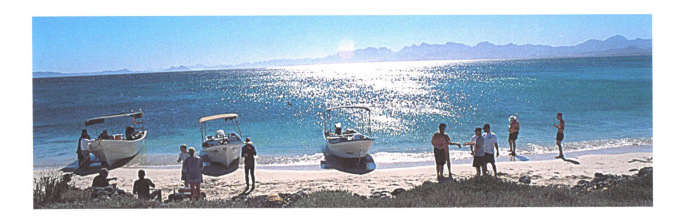

### PIRATES OF THE SEA OF CORTEZ

English privateers left behind a colorful legacy in Baja. In spite of Spain's repeated attempts to colonize the peninsula, the pirates probably gained more wealth in the California's than the Spanish themselves. For 250 years they plagued the Manila galleons off the coast of the California's, finding the bays of Baja's Cape Region perfect hideouts. The most notorious of the Pacific privateers was Sir Thomas Cavendish, whose biggest capture took place at Cabo San Lucas in 1587. After a sea battle, he looted the Spanish galleon Santa Ana, sent its crew and passengers ashore, and then proceeded to set it on fire. The treasure was divided between his two English vessels, Desire and Content. The two ships set sail for England, but during the night the Content disappeared. Cavendish reported in England that the captain and crew must have taken the ship to a nearby island and disappeared with the loot. Neither the wreckage of the vessel nor the treasure was ever discovered. Daniel Defoe's 'Robinson Crusoe' was inspired by the famed pirate Woodes Rogers, when he landed in La Paz after rescuing a seaman who had been marooned 5 years on a deserted island off Chile's coast. The rescued man was named Alexander Selkirk, whose island adventure gave life to Robinson Crusoe. Selkirk was aboard Roger's ship Dover when the crew captured the Spanish galleon Encarnacion off Cabo San Lucas in 1709. He then served as sailing master on the ship's return voyage to England the following year.

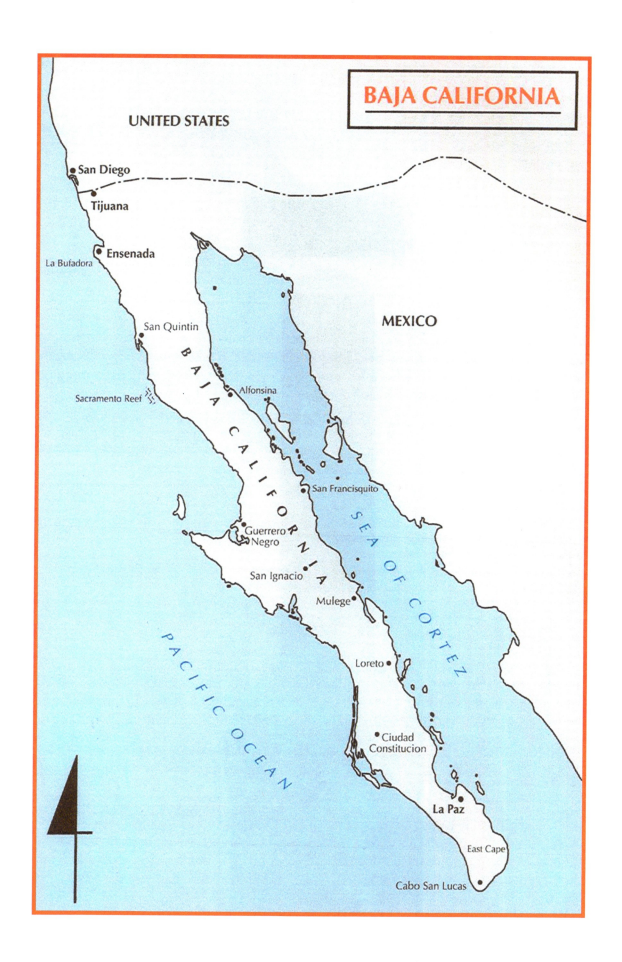

BAJA CALIFORNIA

UNITED STATES

San Diego

Tijuana

Ensenada

La Bufadora

MEXICO

San Quintin

B A J A   C A L I F O R N I A

Sacramento Reef

Alfonsina

San Francisquito

SEA OF CORTEZ

Guerrero Negro

San Ignacio

Mulege

PACIFIC OCEAN

Loreto

Ciudad Constitucion

La Paz

East Cape

Cabo San Lucas

# INFORMATION

**Airlines:** A few commercial airlines fly into Baja. At the present they are; Alaska, Aero California and Aero Mexico. There are daily flights from Los Angeles, San Diego, San Francisco, Phoenix and some of Mexico's major cities. Baja's commercial airports are located in Tijuana, Loreto, La Paz and Los Cabos.

**Driving Tips:** Highway 1 (The Transpeninsular Highway), is a two lane highway. The highway does vary from one section to another. Mountain grades can be quite steep and remote so errors of judgment can have serious consequences. Most of the highway is in good repair but it tends to be narrow in areas and lacks hard shoulders, and curves can be tighter than expected. Trucks in front of you will put on their left blinker when they see that it is clear, telling you it's ok to pass. The blinker does not mean that they are turning left. But always use common sense especially in mountains or blind curves; don't always put your trust in their blinking tail light. You will pass a few military inspection points along the entire peninsula. They are only checking for drugs and firearms. Federales no longer stop and harass tourists. There are Pemex gas stations along the way but it is always a good idea to fill up whenever possible as several areas of Highway 1 has long stretches. Always carry drinking water and watch your speed as many times you may come around a corner only to find range cattle or wild burros crossing the road. Driving at night is not really recommended because of some locals poorly lit vehicles and cattle seeking the warmth of the asphalt, sometimes lying down on the highway. But Baja's grand terrain is truly breathtaking. Gravel roads are normally in reasonable condition, but it depends largely on how long ago they were graded. For the real adventurer, there remain many miles of unpaved roads that will take you about as far from civilization as you would like to go. Four wheel drive is recommended for these off the beaten path roads.

**Insurance:** To be fully protected in Mexico, you must carry Mexican Insurance on your vehicle, trailer and boat. The insurance rates are based on the value and length of your stay. Insurance can be obtained from Auto Club of California or at the border when crossing.

**Currency:** The peso is the unit of exchange but the U.S. dollar is accepted throughout Baja. Usually you can get more for your money by paying in pesos as the vendor does not have to figure out the exchange rate. Banks offer the best exchange rate.

**Entry Requirements:** Birth certificates from United States citizens have been accepted but a passport is highly recommended. It is mandatory on commercial flights. On all flights you will receive a visa aboard the plane. If you are driving you will need to stop at the border to obtain a visa only if you are going further than Guerro Negro, which is halfway down the peninsula. If you forget, you can obtain a visa in Guerro Negro. Citizens from countries other than the United States may need visas in advance.

**Language:** Spanish is the national language although English is spoken quite frequently in the tourist areas. The Spanish spoken in Mexico is Latin American Spanish, unlike the Castilian Spanish spoken in Spain.

**Climate:** Baja's climate ranges from Mediterranean to dry desert, to tropical desert along the Sea of Cortez. Two thirds of the peninsula can be classified as pure desert. Along the Sea of Cortez summer temperatures range from 90-110 degrees F (32-43 degrees C). The weather can get hot and sometimes quite humid. Temperatures cool down in the fall, winter and spring, dropping into the 50'sF (10-15C).

**Electricity:** The electricity is 110 volts, 60 cycles, the same as in the United States.

**Lodging and Food:** The major towns of Tijuana, Ensenada, Mulege, Loreto, La Paz and Cabo San Lucas have a wide variety of hotels and restaurants to choose from. They range from upscale to lower end. The smaller towns in between have motels and tasty little restaurants. While most of the restaurants and hotels serve purified water, if you're not sure, just order bottled.

**Telephone and Internet:** Telephone service is throughout Baja. When dialing from the U.S. to Baja, dial 011-52-area code and number. When dialing from Baja to the U.S. dial 001-area code and number. Phone cards can also be purchased and Internet cafes can be found in all major towns.

**Shopping:** All of the major towns have great little artisan shops including local pottery, ceramics and sterling silver jewelry.

**Time Zone:** Baja Norte (north) is on Pacific Time zone same as the western U.S. states while Baja Sur (south) is in the Mountain Time zone.

**Boat Launch Ramps:** There are launch ramps in all of the major areas of Baja but in remote areas they can be narrow and shallow. Small boats and inflatables do not have much of a problem in launching but for larger boats you will need to launch from major towns. In many of the smaller villages that are accessible by dirt roads, one of the easiest ways for launching small craft is the same as the locals, just launch directly from the shoreline!

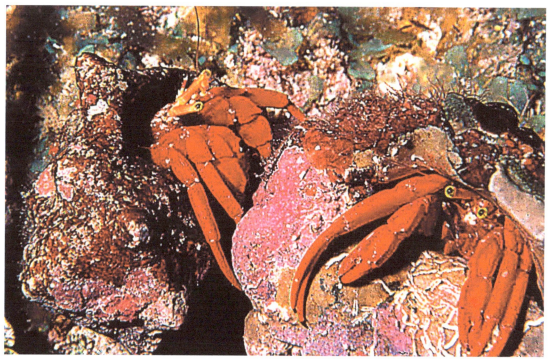

**Redlegged hermit crabs touring the reef at night.**

# Chapter II  THE SEA OF CORTEZ

If you ever wondered where the spectacular Colorado River in the U.S. finally meets the Sea of Cortez, the highway heading south from Mexicali runs within one mile of the Colorado. At this southern location the once mighty Colorado is not much more than a slow moving pond, but it is indeed the same water that runs through Lake Powell, Lake Mead, Lake Mojave and Lake Havasu before it crosses the border into Baja east of Calexico. If you want to see the Colorado River in Baja, just turn left off of Baja Highway 5 at Km. 68 (Yurimuri exit). Go straight one half mile and then straight again on the smaller dirt road where the wider graded road forks to the right. The water you see traveled over 1,000 miles to get here and it is going to continue on for another 1000!

## Diving and Snorkeling

The Sea of Cortez, also known as the Gulf of California is a magnificent body of water that divides Mexico's western mainland and the Baja peninsula. The first 100 miles of this vast sea is in effect a continuation of the Colorado River estuary. This area extends as far south as Puertecitos and is quite shallow, reaching a depth of only 60ft ten miles offshore. The extreme north of this area is the natural spawning grounds of many of the mullet, corvina, white seabass and croaker that live throughout the Sea of Cortez. These shallow waters receive continuous nutrients from the Colorado River to nourish the food chain of plankton and bait fish that feeds the schools of migrating fish that at different times of the year are found throughout the Sea of Cortez.

Beneath the waters of this vast sea, lies a plethora of marine life discoveries. Over 800 varieties of fish have been identified and biologists believe there are at least 3,000 species of marine animals total and many are endemic only to the Sea of Cortez. This sea has acted as a giant fish trap that has collected marine species over many thousands of years from the nearby Pacific, the South Pacific and even the Caribbean (through a now extinct water merge between the two bodies of water). Many of these have evolved into species unique only to the Sea of Cortez. Approximately 90% of these species can be found close to Baja's shores and outer islands. Its 20ft (6m) tides create currents that aerate the water and stir up nutrients, which support a food chain ranging from plankton to giant whales. With the great difference in water temperature throughout the different seasons, the sea has a tremendous amount of migrating marine animals. Twenty five species of whales frequent Baja's sea, including the humpback, gray, finback, minke, sperm, pilot, sei, brydes, goosebeaked, killer whales, false killer whales and dwarf sperm. Commonly seen are bottlenose and Pacific white-sided dolphins, sometimes in pods of thousands. The spotted, spinner, striped and Risso's dolphins also find refuge here as does the small rare vaquita dolphin, endemic only to the northern part of the sea.

Long known for its large pelagics, such as the giant manta rays, whale sharks and hammerhead sharks, over 60 species of sharks have been identified but the scalloped hammerhead is the most common. Somewhat shy, if you are lucky, you can catch a glimpse of one or occasionally several usually gliding over seamounts and around offshore pinnacles. Feeding on fish, these fabulous prehistoric looking creatures are known to school in the thousands. Sadly through the advent of the Asian markets, many of these incredible animals have been caught, had their fins cut off (known as finning), the shark then thrown back into the water only to die a slow agonizing death. Global education of the true importance in the role that sharks play in our oceans ecosystem will be their only hope for future survival.

The barren islands of the Sea of Cortez are as beautiful topside as they are underwater. These grandly sculptured land formations are home to rabbits, reptiles, rodents and thousands of seabirds. These include;

the graceful frigate, blue-footed booby, brown booby, masked booby, brown pelican, egret, cormorant, blue heron, sandpiper and ten species of gull. Another furry little resident is the California sea lion. They can be seen dozing in the sun along island shores or frolicking swiftly past you underwater.

But one thing is for sure; wherever your ventures take you along this grand peninsula, a world of discovery awaits…

## Underwater Environment:
There are four main types of underwater habitats in the Sea of Cortez. They are reefs, walls, seamounts and sandy bottoms.

### Reefs:
Every island has reef structures whether volcanically formed or not. Some of the reefs are made up of huge boulders where they seem as if some giant fitted them together like a massive puzzle. Boulders do a balancing act, forming caverns, grottos, overhangs and jagged crevices. Reef fishes inhabit all of the reefs, but in some locations you will find more of certain species. Typically seen are the bright blue and gold king angels, the gray and yellow cortez angels, surgeonfish, barberfish, colorful wrasses, triggerfish, damselfish, sergeant majors, a variety of eels in all sizes, Mexican hogfish, trumpetfish, pufferfish and groupers. Most of the reef structures begin quite shallow sloping gradually to deeper depths. Around the offshore islets where reef crests break the surface, schools of snapper, jacks and yellowtail can be found. The leeward side of these outer islets harbor beautiful fan shaped gorgonian corals of brightly colored reds, yellows and oranges. The reefs rocky substrate is home to a plethora of invertebrates. Starfish seem to come in every variety. Some have very thick bodies and arms, while others have long spindly arms. Their sizes vary and their colors range from deep purple to bright orange to bright yellow to being covered with spines and even some having the appearance of a chocolate chip cookie.

### Walls:
Most of the offshore islands have areas where walls flow steeply, only interrupted by jagged ledges, and then continue down into deeper water of over 100ft. (30m). The steeper sides are frequently covered with seafans and gorgonian corals. As currents are usually stronger along walls, the corals open up to feed on the flowing nutrients. Tiny brilliantly colored nudibranchs can be found foraging. The golden colored black coral bushes can be seen as shallow as 60ft (18m). Some of Baja's greater walls can be found around the East Cape and Cabo San Lucas where the submarine canyon drops dramatically into the abyss. Walls are beautiful dives and on drift dives you can easily just flow with the current if there is one. Larger fish along with blue water pelagics are more frequently seen in these areas.

### Seamounts:
Seamounts are awesome places to dive. They are literally the tops of submerged mountains. They are generally deeper dives, often starting around 50ft (15m). The peaks of these mounts have the usual undercuts and crevices of most reef systems. But because of the deep water upwelling around them, they have a more vast variety of marine life. One usually finds more turtles, moray eels, fish schools, including the roosterfish, Pacific amberjack and pompanos.

The sloping walls of these great peaks drop rapidly into the blue. In the 80 to 100ft (24-36m) range is where divers are more likely to encounter great manta rays, large tuna, wahoo, hammerhead sharks and on lucky occasions, giant whale sharks, swordfish, marlin and sailfish.

### Sandy Bottoms:
Many times divers don't imagine sandy bottoms as being great dives, but in the right area they can make for incredible dives. Sandy bottoms are found at the base of all reefs and offshore from sandy beaches. Because of the wide open space, the inhabitants here are masters of disguise. Flatfish such as flounder, halibut, turbot and sand dabs are found camouflaged on the bottom. Large stingrays, graceful spotted eagle rays, angel sharks, oversized bullseye pufferfish, schools of goatfish, grunts and mullet can be seen foraging across this flat surface. A variety of shellfish including, the horse conch, an array of clams and several types of beautifully colored anemones make their homes within this grainy environment.

**Water Temperature:** The Sea of Cortez has the largest water temperature change than any other sea. The summer and early fall months, mid-June to late October brings in warm water of temperatures into the low and mid 80'sF (29-30C). A 3mm wetsuit is recommended not only for warmth but for protection from tiny stinging buggers that can float on the surface certain times of the year. In November and December the temperature drops into the 70'sF (22-28C), while the months from January through May the water usually fluctuates in the mid 60'sF (16–20C). A 5mm-7mm wetsuit is recommended and a hood is also a good idea.

**Weather:** In the northern section of Baja, the weather is much like Southern California. Winters can be chilly with wind and rain. The summer season is balmier. Southern Baja does get occasional tropical storms that can last a few days. Chubascos are local warm winds with thunderstorms, prevalent from June through October. Hurricanes do happen occasionally mostly affecting Baja's tip around the Cabo San Lucas area. These storms bring visibility down and other areas of the sea will feel its affect. The local fishermen know about weather conditions, so if you are exploring Baja with your own boat, keep an eye on what they are doing. Ask their opinion; which if not in the scientific statistics, is more than likely quite reliable.

**Currents:** Certain dive sites can have currents. It is a good idea to check with your Divemaster, if on a boat or locals if exploring on your own. Currents can pick up in certain areas especially along the points, walls and seamounts. Currents can also be stronger on full and new moons. Always remember the standard rule; swim against the current at the beginning of your dive and with it coming back, unless it is a drift dive, where a planned boat will pick you up.

**Visibility:** Visibility can vary depending on location, but on calm days it can reach 100ft (30m) plus. During the winter months plankton blooms happen which lessen the visibility but this also brings in the whales, which feed on them so whale watching is at its best. Depending on conditions, snorkelers have on occasion been able to interact with these gentle giants. The summer and fall months usually have the highest visibility.

**Boat Diving:** In the larger towns of Mulege, Loreto, La Paz, East Cape and Cabo San Lucas, there are dive shops with charter boats available. Commonly used are pangas, (a fast smaller Mexican boat). Several islands sit offshore from Mulege, Loreto and La Paz which offer good dive sites. If you plan to drive down with your own boat, inflatables and small boats are excellent for offshore reefs and some close by islets. Larger boats with longer range are needed for the outer islands.

**Shore Diving:** There is some good diving along the shoreline. The best areas would be around rocky points. These are also good areas for snorkeling. But remember, sandy bottoms make for pretty cool dives as well.

**Dive Equipment:** The larger towns do have dive shops with rental equipment, but sometimes when it was last serviced can be a question. Be sure that it is a reputable shop with tanks that have hydrostatic tests and visual inspections up to date. Bringing your own personal gear is always a plus. Most dive shops provide tanks and weights in their charter price.

**Night Diving:** Several hours after sunset, the underwater world undergoes a remarkable transformation. A host of nocturnal animals which hide in the daylight hours become very active. It is a great opportunity to get photographs of fish as they lie sleepily on the bottom and in crevices. You will find the parrotfish all wrapped up in a white silky looking cocoon which he makes every night for bedtime. A protective wrap, by morning he will roll it up into a ball, discarding it on the reef. Moray eels and lobster can be seen moving across the reef in search of food. The darkness also brings an amazing variety of invertebrates out. Flowering golden cup corals will blanket the overhangs as octopus crawl atop their ledges, and the sandy bottom begins to come alive with the snake-like bodies of the 3ft long (1m) synapted cucumbers. And the reef pockets are stuffed with colored anemones and tiny red shrimp.

**Snorkeling:** There are many opportunities for snorkelers. Almost any beach with rocky outcroppings makes for good snorkeling. Shallow reefs are usually prolific with life. The offshore islands can be great as well as the shallow tops of walls. Seamounts can be deep but snorkeling over them has its plus side. In blue water snorkeling is where we have seen sailfish, mantas and schools of fish as there are no scuba bubbles to frighten them off.

**Conservation:** As with so many oceans of our world today, Mexico's waters are up against the same problems. Although the Mexican government still has a ways to go in order to protect its greatest asset; the Sea of Cortez is still quite prolific. Some of the main problems it has faced have been illegal fishing and gill nets, which have become the scourge of the sea. Foreign fish markets have been its biggest enemy. The process has been slow but with stronger restrictions and regulations coming into affect, the hope of the future gleams brighter. Several areas have now been made into national underwater parks, where no game can be taken within certain boundaries. For visitors to take any game they must have a Mexican fishing license and certain game is prohibited.

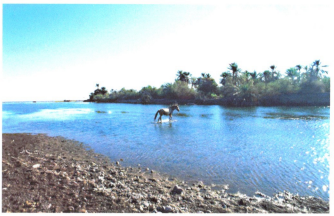

**Animals roam freely in the estuaries.**

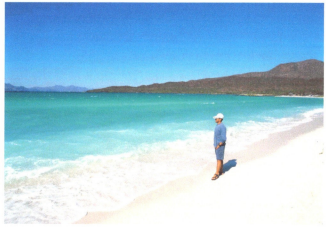

**Looking out from Coronado Is. towards Loreto.**

# Chapter III   ALFONSINA

*A Baja reality reminder... 'You can't depend on your judgment when your imagination is out of focus'*
*(Mark Twain)*

**About The Area:** Not having changed much from past generations, this area consists of small fishing communities. Surrounding Alfonsina's pristine coastline, foreign owned vacation homes are popping up. Gonzaga Bay is a beautiful and pristine area. It has been a gringo getaway since John Wayne discovered the place while on holiday between western movie shoots. The fact that it is so difficult to get to has a lot to do with its slow growth. Bahia de Gonzaga is approximately 100 miles south of San Felipe, and about 45 tough miles south of Puertecitos. The road south from Puertecitos has long had a reputation for being one of the worst roads in Baja. Despite the significant road grading provided by the Mexican government in the 1980's, this road is still very intimidating to all but the most seasoned Baja traveler. This area actually consists of two separate bays, connected by a small tidal flow at higher tides, and a shallow sand bar at low tide. The large front bay faces the Sea of Cortez, and tends to be the main bay for most activities and the back bay is almost fully protected, except for a wide access channel just up from Papa Fernandez Camp on the north end.

**Getting There:** Getting to Alfonsina can be quite an adventure for those that are driving. There is a rough 45 mile (73 km) dirt road coming from the north. As with most dirt roads throughout Baja, four wheel drive is recommended. It is always a good idea to bring food, water and ice. There is another road just south of Catavina and north of Chapala off Highway 1. It is approximately 40 miles (65km) and is on a somewhat better dirt road. Some visitors fly in by small private planes. The old dirt airstrip runs north/south and is conveniently located by the water. The only drawback is it gets flooded during high tide. The newer hard packed Rancho Grande airstrip runs east/west, from the beach to the main highway. This airstrip is very long, and is in excellent condition. A landing fee may be charged.

**Accommodations:** **Alfonsina's Resort** is located near the end of the sand spit at the north end of the dirt runway. It has 16 rooms, a restaurant and a bar on the beach.

**Camping:** There are many places along the shore, both north and south of Gonzaga bay, where a Baja traveler can set up camp on open beaches. In addition, there are three areas to camp which offer some degree of services. **Papa Fernandez Camp**, turn west off the main gravel road at the sign. **Alfonsina's Resort** is a mile or so past **Papa's.** Sandy beaches await your tent near the restaurant and bathrooms and showers are available for a modest fee. **Rancho Grande Camp** has palapas with toilets at the waters edge. Taking the gravel road from the main road, at the intersection where the market and Pemex station intersect, it is one mile south of **Alphonsina's.**

**Launch Ramps:** There is a boat launching ramp at **Papa Fernandez**, through the village to the right. Also, launching near **Alphonsina's** behind the old airstrip (at high tide). Small boats and inflatables can easily be launched from the sandy shoreline.

**Diving & Snorkeling:** There are no diving facilities, but local fishermen are usually willing to take people out in their pangas for a fee.

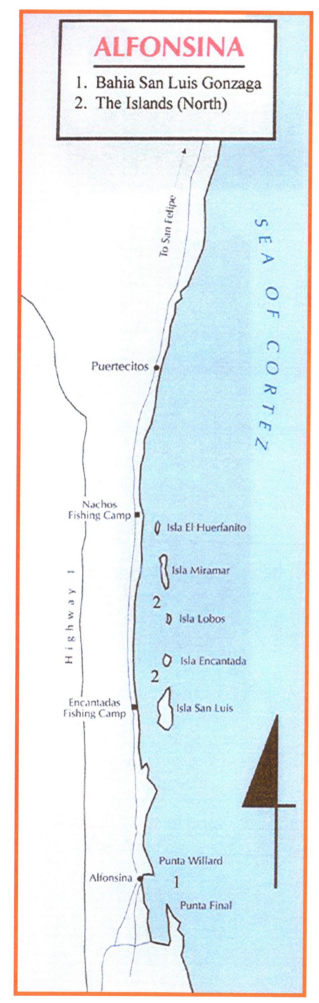

## ALFONSINA

1. Bahia San Luis Gonzaga
2. The Islands (North)

To San Felipe

SEA OF CORTEZ

Puertecitos

Highway 1

Nachos
Fishing Camp

2  Isla El Huerfanito

Isla Miramar

2  Isla Lobos

Isla Encantada

2
Encantadas
Fishing Camp        Isla San Luis

Punta Willard

Alfonsina        1

Punta Final

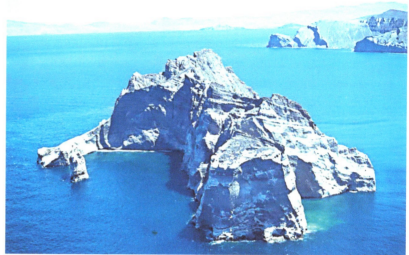

**One of the desolate islands between Alfonsina and Puertecitos**

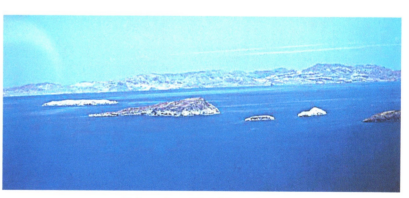

**Islands off Alfonsina.**

11

## 1.  BAHIA SAN LUIS GONZAGA

**THE DEPTH** range is approximately 10-40ft (3-12m) and the diving is accessible by either shore or boat. Alfonsina is encompassed by a large bay and the surrounding shoreline is dotted with rocky outcroppings, which make excellent snorkeling spots. Just off the point to the north, the rocky substrate stair steps its way down to a sandy bottom to a depth of about 40ft (12m). A variety of reef fish find refuge here. Convict tangs, bright green parrotfish, cartoon looking tiny boxfish, filefish, black durgon and sergeant majors are just some of what you will most likely see. Several types of invertebrates such as seastars, urchins and anemones can be found clinging to the reef. The bay is also a playground for local sea lions that you sometimes see zipping around in the shallows. This area on occasion has brought in the giant whale sharks. Usually spotted in late spring or early summer, these passive plankton eating sharks almost seem oblivious to the presence of divers and snorkelers. Following the rocky coastline from Alfonsina's to Cactus Point one will find many places to enjoy and explore.

## 2.  THE ISLANDS (North)

**THE DEPTH** ranges from 15-100+ ft (5-30+m) and these four islands are located about 10 miles north of Alfonsina and sit a couple of miles offshore. They are only accessible by boat. The islands are made up of a hard substrate with dramatic steep walls. Detached rocks surround the islands which are quite interesting to explore. The water is shallow close to the island but then drops dramatically into deeper depths. In these shallow grooves, snorkelers can find a lot to see. A variety of reef fish and invertebrate life surround the rocky outcroppings. Divers will usually encounter grouper, cabrilla and snapper along with smaller reef fish and rays. The entire island chain runs about 12 miles (19km) and Isla San Luis is the closest and the largest of the chain. The three islands north of this are, Isla Encantada, Isla Lobos and Isla Miramar. Because of the great tidal change in the Baja Norte, the visibility is usually low, about 20-30ft (6-9m).

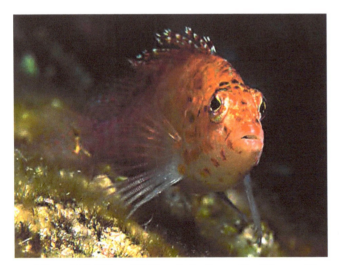

**About 3.5 in. (8.5cm) in length, the red coral hawkfish lives throughout the reefs.**

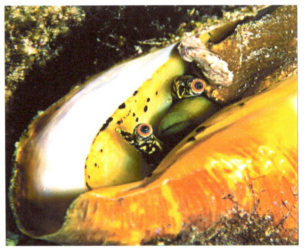

**About 10 in. (250mm) long, a curious cortez conch peeks out from its shell.**

# Chapter IV   BAHIA DE LOS ANGELES

*A Baja reality reminder... 'Attitude is more important than facts'*
*(Karl Menniger)*

**About The Area:** Bahia de Los Angeles was discovered in 1746 by Jesuit Father Fernando Consag. This attempt was to find an easier and faster way to the Sea of Cortez to supply the missionaries that occupied the San Francisco de Borja Mission, which was located on the top of a mountain 35 kilometers from the bay.

This 12 mile long bay is probably one of the most picturesque bays on the Sea of Cortez. The coastline is made up of miles of white sandy beaches while the bay is studded with islands. At one time this area was a productive turtle fishing region, but over harvesting has led to their decline. At the north edge of town there is a small protected turtle conservation and research center which is an effort to bring these grand creatures back to fruition. Visitors are welcome and donations are greatly appreciated. The town is a fun place to explore. There is a small museum behind the town's central plaza which has gold and silver mining exhibits, fossils, whale skeletons and Indian artifacts. Mining once played a big part in Bahia de Los Angeles history. The toy-like locomotive in front of the museum was once used on the mines. The local mines of Santa Marta and San Juan produced gold and silver in the 1800's. You can still see a smelter and the old jail. One of the mines railway is 11 miles (18km) south of the bay and Santa Marta is reached by hiking only, so plan a day trip for an interesting hike up to the old mine.

**Getting There:** There are no major airlines that fly into Bahia de Los Angeles, however, there are two runways for small aircraft. If driving, from Highway 1, there is a sign pointing to a 41 mile (66 km) paved road from Punta Prieta that leads to the bay. The paved road does end once you reach the town of Bahia de Los Angeles so it is a good idea to have a dependable dirt road vehicle if you plan to do much exploring beyond.

**Accommodations:** There are several motels to stay at. In town, there are the **Las Hamacas**, **Villa Vitta, Costa del Sol, Guillermos** on the beach and a little south is **Casa Diaz.** All are clean with fair prices. For more upscale accommodations there is **Los Vientas Spa and Resort** and **Villa Bahia**, north of town.

**Camping:** You can camp almost anywhere along the coastline on your own. If you are looking for a remote area with scenic and spectacular views, you'll find it at Punta Gringa, about 25 minutes north of town on the coast. But for camping amenities, **Camp Gecko** is located 4 miles south of town on the water. They offer palapas and camping cabins which have toilets and hot showers. North of town is **Daggett's Campground** which has palapas and casitas available with toilets, hot showers, a small restaurant and store. Also **Raquel and Larry's** have camping accommodations and rooms.

**Launch Ramps:** The **Casa Diaz ramp** is concrete, 14 ft. (4.2m) wide and has a small breakwater. Check with the office before launching. The **Villa Vitta ramp** is 12 ft. (3.6m) wide and is concrete and can be used at high or low tide. Check with Villa Vitta Motel before launching. There is also another ramp in front of **Guillermos's trailer park.**

**Diving Facilities:** Both **Daggetts Campground** and **Camp Gecko** have air compressors to fill tanks and do take divers out in their boats.

**Diving and Snorkeling:** Bahia de Los Angeles is dotted with offshore islands and is extremely picturesque. These offshore islands make for some great dive sites and all easily reached by boat. Early morning dives are recommended because this bay is notorious for its strong afternoon winds which blow out of the canyons west of town. The water temperatures tend to stay cooler here ranging from 65F (18C) in the winter months to 75F (27C) in summer and early fall. Currents from deep canyons are being forced to the surface by the extreme tidal ranges in this area. Tidal currents reach their maximum during full and new moons. It is a good idea to consider moon phases and tidal changes when planning your dives. For drift dives you can take advantage of the stronger currents as long as there is an experienced person in a boat, following your bubbles.

Different species of fish move in and out of this area according to the seasons. At certain times of the year snapper, sierra mackerel, yellowtail and halibut can be seen. Many year round fish, such as bass and grouper can reach tremendous sizes around the outer offshore islands. The colorful reef fish hang around the reefs all year round. The big channel between the largest island which is Isla Angel de La Guarda and the closer islands is safe harbor to sea lion rookeries, manta rays, dolphins and several species of migrating whales. Seasonally, whale sharks have come into the bay to feed when there are large plankton blooms. These shallow waters provide both food and protection.

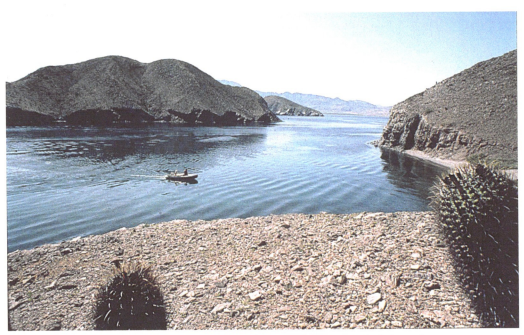

**Bahia de Los Angeles is studded with islands.**

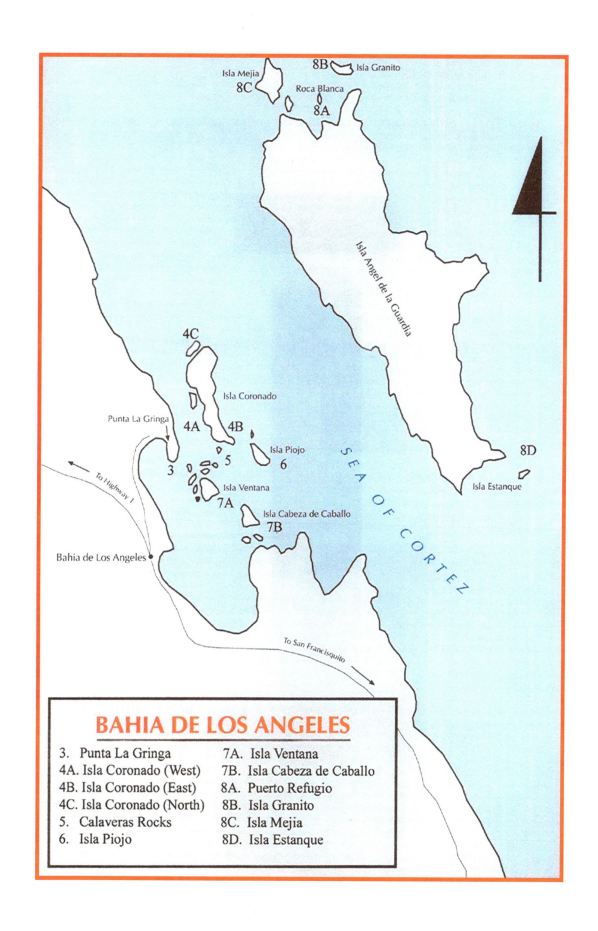

**BAHIA DE LOS ANGELES**

3. Punta La Gringa
4A. Isla Coronado (West)
4B. Isla Coronado (East)
4C. Isla Coronado (North)
5. Calaveras Rocks
6. Isla Piojo

7A. Isla Ventana
7B. Isla Cabeza de Caballo
8A. Puerto Refugio
8B. Isla Granito
8C. Isla Mejia
8D. Isla Estanque

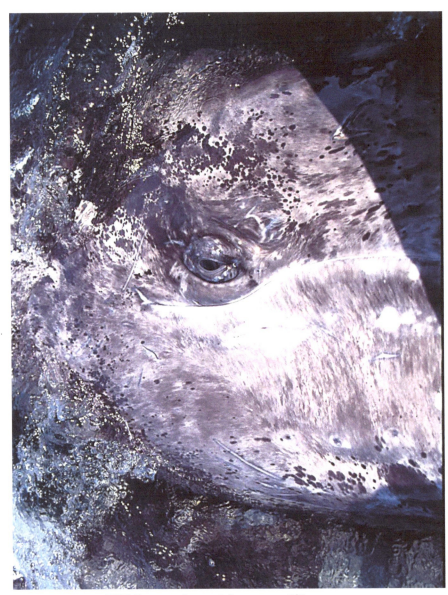

**With an almost human-like eye,
a gray whale surfaces to look around.**

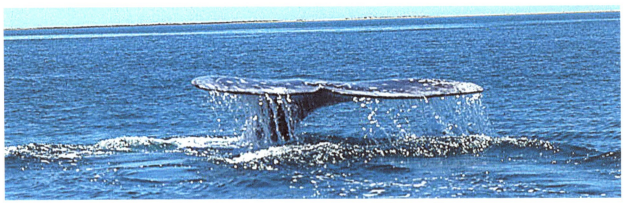

**After visiting, a gray whale takes a dive.**

## 3. PUNTA LA GRINGA

**THE DEPTH** is in the 10-30ft (3-9m) range and for the most part it is a sandy bottom with cobble rocks and small reef patches. Punta la Gringa is the point just north of the Bay and is usually protected against wave action. It is a good snorkeling area for finding shellfish, flatfish and various tropical fish. Bahia de Los Angeles itself is a massive area of white sand. In these somewhat shallow bay waters, divers can find chocolate clams, tiger paw and bay scallops and occasionally horse conch. This granular environment can actually make for some very interesting dives. Stingrays and flatfish are commonly seen as are occasional angel sharks. Large bullseye pufferfish will linger slightly above the bottom as sea stars, sea pens and burrowing anemones make homes in the sandy pockets along the bottom. Look closely, sometimes you will see the head of a spotted snake eel poking up out of the sand; when frightened, he will quickly sink back into the sand, his hole caving in and then 'whoosh', vanishing. And once again the sand becomes what appears to be, a lifeless flat bottom.

## 4. ISLA CORONADO

**THE DEPTH** around this island ranges from 15-90+ ft (5-27+ m). Isla Coronado is also known as Isla Smith and is 4 miles (6.5 km) in length. Near the south end of Coronado, on the **West side (4A)**, there is an extensive lagoon "Rada Laguna" and south of this is a protected bay. There is some pretty good snorkeling around the rocky outcroppings. Directly across the cobble bar from the lagoon at Rada Laguna on the **East side (4B)** of the island is another large bay. The south shore is loaded with rocks and reefs and these detached rocks begin from the middle of the island extending to the southern tip. This east side is typical of the Sea of Cortez. Large boulders teeter on each other, spilling onto colorful reef structures. The reef in this area starts at about 15ft (5m) dropping gradually to over 90ft (27m). This rocky terrain has crevices and small chimneys which give way to streams of flickering sunlight. In the deeper crevices you will find schools of bright orange glasseyes, soldierfish and cardinalfish, which spend most of their lives in the darker pockets of the reefs.

One interesting little critter is the mauve-colored flower urchin. It has short pedal-like appendages that ripple slowly along the flatter spots picking up tiny pieces of shells to wear. At first glance these little guys just appear to be a small pile of broken shells. There are many other colorful invertebrates, such as bright colored feather duster worms, a variety of shellfish and an array of sea stars including the crown of thorns. Look closely at the underarms of the sea stars; a tiny pinkish parasitic cup shell about 0.5in.(12mm) in length lives here. The larger female shell covers the smaller male, and both get nourishment by sucking fluids from their sea star host. Surrounding these rocky substrates are many reef fishes, such as the polka dotted guinea puffers, cortez chubs, a variety of wrasses and soapfish. Soapfish have brown bodies with white blotches and live in crevices in the daylight hours, but come out at night to feed. If touched, they give off a protective soapy film that their bodies secrete which is a toxin to other fish.

At the **North End (4C)** of Isla Coronado, there is a small islet called **Isla Coronadito** which is separated from the island by a deep narrow channel. The islet is characterized by its sharp drop-offs. Larger fish such as a variety of jacks, yellowtail and grouper are more prevalent around these drop-offs because of the swifter currents which bring up nutrients and food from the deep water upwelling.

On the north and west side of this islet the water is about 20ft (6m) in depth with a gradual slope. This is a good area for both snorkeling and scuba diving. Large rocks dominate the terrain which gives protection to reef fishes and invertebrates that make their homes in the scattered fissures below.

## 5. CALAVERAS ROCKS

**THE DEPTH** around these rocks is in the 30-40ft (9-12m) range. Known to the locals as Sea Lion Rock, these offshore structures are located at the southern end of Isla Coronado a half mile out (.8 km). Surrounding these rocks the depths are quite shallow and continue deeper with a gradual slope. There is a sea lion colony that hangs out here which always makes for a great dive when these curious playful clowns swim around you, occasionally grabbing your fins or harassing you in some friendly way. They will speed up, stopping inches from your mask, blow bubbles, and then dart away. At certain times of the year the large bulls can become aggressive, particularly when new pups have arrived. They will give a fair warning with an underwater bark showing their teeth, at which time it is best to respect their wishes and give them their space.

Fish life, shellfish and beautiful shades of purple, red, white and orange gorgonian sea fans are sprinkled along the sides of these rocks slowly waving in rhythm to the water movement.

## 6.  ISLA PIOJO

**THE DEPTH** surrounding this island runs in the 30-40ft (9-12m) range. Isla Piojo sits just southeast of Coronado Island. There are large rocky formations scattered around the points. The bottom terrain is sand with huge boulders, which makes for good snorkeling and shallow diving. Depending on the season, great balls consisting of thousands of baitfish will cloud up the water. Their movement creates streaks of flickering silver as they move through the fluid sunrays. These fish balls bring in larger fish that frequent the area. Roosterfish and corvina are local habitants. There is a cabbage-like algae that grows in the bay and among the rocks, attracting invertebrates which feed on it. Gorgeous nudibranchs decorated with frills of green, navy, yellow, orange, red, purple, white and polka dots can be found needling their way through the undergrowth. Many times nudibranchs are found where there is more current which carries nutrients.

## 7. ISLA VENTANA and ISLA CABEZA DE CABALLO

**THE DEPTH** around these inner islands is in the 15-60+ ft (5-18+ m) range. There are a few clustered islets that dot the inner bay but the two main islands closest to the town of Bahia de Los Angeles are **Isla Ventana (7A)** and **Isla Cabeza De Caballo (7B)**, both of which are great areas for scuba diving and snorkeling. The shallow waters along their shores have a gradual decline in depth and are lined with rocky boulders and river type rocks. There is a reef between them known as Marcelo. This area harbors an abundance of shellfish including the large pen scallop that can reach up to over one foot (31cm) in length. It buries itself where just the upper portion protrudes above the sand. Amazingly though, as large as this shell gets, the little animal inside is quite small. Reef fishes are more sporadic. Schools of yellowtail and jacks are more often seen from December to June, while October through April brings in more snapper and roosterfish. Tropicals such as the king and cortez angelfish, barberfish, surgeonfish, Mexican hogfish and wrasses are seen around these rocky outcroppings year round.

## 8.  ISLA ANGEL DE LA GUARDA

**THE DEPTH** around this island varies but in most areas it is 20-100+ ft (6-30+ m). This island is the largest of the offshore islands and is the furthest out. Angel de La Guarda sits 20 miles (32 km) out from Bahia de Los Angeles and the north end is actually 40 miles (65 km) from the bay. This 42 mile (68 km) long stretch of land with its 4000 ft (1212 m) high mountains makes it a prominent landmark. It is home to a variety of life including rodents, lizards, coyotes and many sea birds. **Puerto Refugio (8A)** is at the north end of the island and has good anchorage from weather. The almost surrealistic pinnacles of white and black rocks, protruding from the water's surface form the most majestic backdrop. These isolated reefs begin in about 30ft (9m) of water and slope down to deeper depths which provide outstanding diving. Schooling jacks, yellowtail, cabrilla, triggerfish, pargo and grouper frequent this entire area along with a menagerie of colorful reef fish. Night dives are great and divers may see all four types of lobster that live in the Sea of Cortez. They are the socorro, the blue spiny, the California spiny and the slipper lobster, all being very tasty.

There is a large pinnacle approximately a half mile (.8 km) offshore from Puerto Refugio. It is surrounded by a rock covered ledge about 40ft (12m) deep. Continuing out there is a series of sharp walls that stair step down to around 90ft (27m). The marine life in this area is very abundant.

**Isla Granito (8B)** is a small islet that sits beyond the pinnacle. A few hundred yards off its northwest side is a reef that starts at a depth of 40ft (12m) and drops to 70ft (21m) to a sandy bottom with scattered rocks. Swaying gorgonians, stinging white hydroids and various sponges cover the hard substrate. Larger schools of fish seem to hang out here along with the big bumphead parrotfish, azure parrotfish, cortez and king angelfish, cortez chubs and cabrilla just to name a few. This area is quite rich with marine invertebrate life as well.

**Isla Mejia (8C)** is a small islet defined with saw cut cliffs and is located on the west side of Puerto Refugio. The north side is excellent for macro photography when the water is calm. An assortment of anemones, nudibranchs, hermit crabs and a rainbow of spiral worms cover the underwater terrain. There are both rocks that break the surface and submerged rocks that make up a reef which extends for over half a mile (.8 km), many of which make for great dive sites.

**Isla Estanque (8D)** is an islet located at the southeast end of La Guarda, where a long reef is connected. The south end of the island is also the closest anchorage from the town of Bahia de Los Angeles. The detached rocks off its shore are an excellent spot for snorkeling. For diving, the depth starts at 40ft (12m) and drops rapidly to hundreds of feet. Estanque's east side has a steep wall with overhangs which makes it an excellent place to explore. The many nooks and crannies are filled with shellfish, including the pink murex, cowries, bay scallops and spiny oysters. And don't forget to look closely on the sandy bottom, chocolate clams can be found just beneath a thin layer of sand along with conch and resting halibuts. In deeper waters divers have more chances of seeing manta rays, sharks, and tuna and on excitingly rare occasions, beautiful billfish such as marlin, swordfish and sailfish.

Going across the channel from Bahia de Los Angeles to Angel de La Guarda, sightings of a variety of dolphins and whales are frequently seen. Whales include the gray, minke, finback, humpback, pilot, orcas and the giant blue whale. The very large finback whale, which reaches a length of 70ft (21m) is usually found here in the summer months and is the most commonly seen.

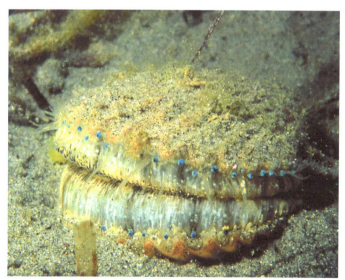

**The calico scallop can easily swim away from predators by jet propulsion.**

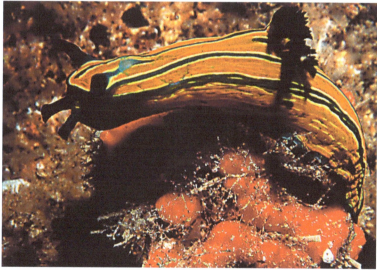

**From 3-12 in. (75-300mm) long, the sea tiger slug swallows nudibranchs whole with hook-like teeth.**

# Chapter V     SAN FRANCISQUITO

**About The Area:**   San Francisquito is a well protected bay located 83 miles (134 km) by land and 50 miles (81 km) by sea south of Bahia de Los Angeles. It offers the most sheltered small boat launching conditions in the entire Midriff area. At the west end you will find a nice white sand beach and there are caves to explore up the two valleys that back the beach. The head of the inner harbor is a beach backed by some vacation cottages. There are limited supplies and gasoline here so come prepared. In the small ranch community of El Barrill, just south of San Francisquito some provisions can be purchased.

**Getting There:**   From Highway 1 there is a turnoff for San Francisquito (look for El Arco sign) about 16.7 miles (27 km) south of the Guerrero Negro junction. From the turnoff, the 75 mile (121 km) road to the bay takes three to four hours, including the steep downgrade known as Cuesta de la Ley (Slope of the Law), which comes along approximately 18 miles (29 km) before San Francisquito.  Nowadays the grade has been lessened and is not quite as challenging as it once was.  Modest supplies may be available along the way in El Arco, 21 miles (33.8 km) east of Highway 1.  Many signless roads join the main one east of El Arco, and you may have to ask directions along the way to ensure you're on a direct course for San Francisquito.

You can also reach San Francisquito by road from Bahia de Los Angeles in about the same amount of time. Between the main street and the small museum, is the road which will lead you there. The road passes through the Sierra San Borja, where there are several impressive ancient Indian petroglyph sites. You can inquire at local ranches for trail guides. Count on lots of washboard along either road; be sure to gas up first in Bahia de Los Angeles, Guerrero Negro or Vizcaino. Both roads meet near Rancho El Progresso, approximately 13 miles (21 km) from Bahia San Francisquito. The network of roads surrounding the ranch can be a trifle confusing; take the branch heading due east to reach the bay (a southeasterly branch goes to the fish camp of El Barril). It is best to have four-wheel drive. San Francisquito also has a small dirt airstrip for small private planes.

**Accommodations:**   There are not a lot of choices here. But, **Resort San Francis Quito** maintains five clean simple, thatched-roof cabanas with cot beds and blankets right on the beach and there are restroom and shower facilities. The resort also offers guest breakfast and dinner.

**Camping:**   The desolate coastline is open for camping but **Alberto & Debra** also allow visitors to camp on their bayside property.  For a little added adventure, they can arrange guided mule trips into the coastal mountain range which is always a fun side trip. You can also purchase fuel and food supplies from them for your own exploration of the area. The **Resort San Francis Quito** permits camping on their grounds which include hot water showers and restrooms.

**Diving Facilities:**   Pangas are available for hire where you can arrange to go out to the local islands. There is a compressor and rental tanks are available, but it is recommended that you bring your own regulators.

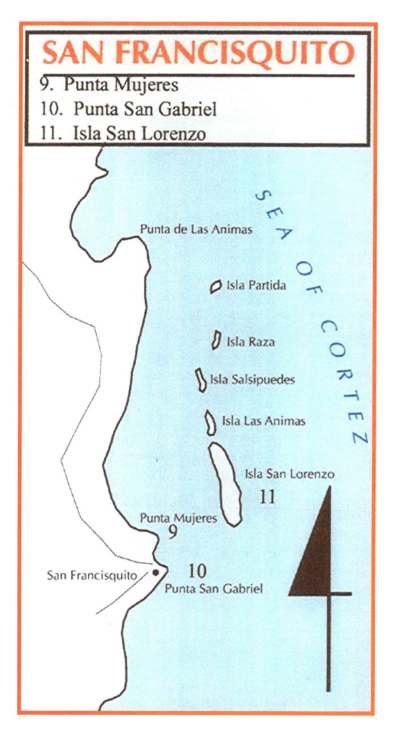

# SAN FRANCISQUITO

9. Punta Mujeres
10. Punta San Gabriel
11. Isla San Lorenzo

Punta de Las Animas

Isla Partida

Isla Raza

Isla Salsipuedes

Isla Las Animas

Isla San Lorenzo

11

Punta Mujeres

9

San Francisquito

10

Punta San Gabriel

SEA OF CORTEZ

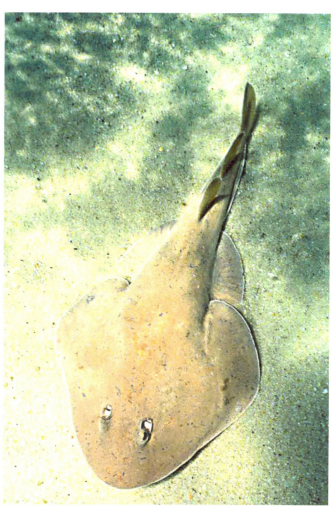

**The electric ray grows to about 3ft ((0.9m) in length. It's a nocturnal animal, feeding on various type worms.**

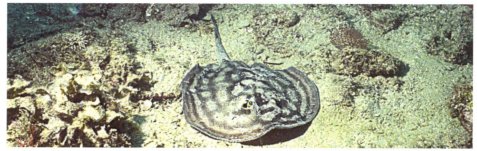

**The bullseye stingray feeds on crabs and worms.**

## 9.  PUNTA MUJERES

THE DEPTH off of Punta Mujeres is around 6-10ft (2-3m) and has a very gradual slope to deeper depths. This point sits to the north of the bay and is decorated with scattered rocks. It is an ideal place to snorkel and can also be quite interesting for shallow scuba dives. In the summer months it is common to see schools of mobulas which is a smaller version of the giant manta ray. These little guys reach a width of about 6ft (1.8m) and hang around rocky outcroppings. Being plankton feeders they glide through the water like some type of majestic looking alien aircraft. An array of reef fish live throughout including damsels, angelfish, blennies and gobies. The rocks are also alive with a variety of invertebrates.

## 10.  PUNTA SAN GABRIEL

THE DEPTH off of Punta San Gabriel is around 6-10ft (2-3m) and is also a good area for snorkeling and shallow dives. This point sits south of the bay. Large boulders litter the bottom as it slopes seaward to open sand where a variety of flatfish, including rays, angel sharks and halibut camouflage themselves. Around the tips of the points currents can really kick up, but if you stay inside of the points, the water is usually calm. You can drive over to both Punta Mujeres and Punta San Gabriel, or you can hike there, which is about a half mile (.8 km) either way. There are easy entries from both shores with rarely any surf to speak of and the beaches are pristine and desolate.

## 11.  ISLA SAN LORENZO

THE DEPTH at Isla San Lorenzo ranges from about 50-100+ ft (15-30+m) and this is the largest of the islands in the chain north of the bay, extending over 10 miles (16 km) in length. It is also the closest to the bay of San Francisquito. Most diving along the submerged cliffs start at about 50ft (15m). Diving is excellent when the sea is calm and the turbidity is down. Because of the tidal currents which push up deep nutrient rich water, the water around the island is usually cool. The depth drops rapidly, plummeting to hundreds of feet. Currents can get very strong so this area is recommended for experienced divers. But this is the place to find larger fish. In the winter and spring months there are a variety of bass and schools of yellowtail. There is no feeling that is more surrealistic than being enveloped within a school of thousands of fish, be it jacks, Mexican barracuda or even baitfish. The summer months bring in groupers, yellowfin tuna, dorado and the humboldt squid. The ledges and deep ravines are home to pargo, snapper and cabrilla along with a myriad of reef fish.

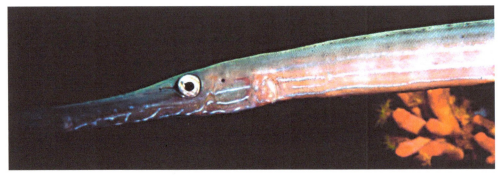

**The trumpetfish often swims beside larger fish, using them
to approach small fish and crustaceans.**

# Chapter VI    MULEGE

*A Baja reality reminder... 'Some of the world's greatest feats were accomplished by people not smart enough to know they were impossible'*

(Doug Larson)

**About The Area:**    The town of Mulege, with a population of 6,000 + is a palm tree lined oasis. The Rio Santa Rosalia is an estuary river that meanders lazily through the valley, finally weaving its way around to meet the waters of the Sea of Cortez. The town is spread out on both banks of the river, a couple miles up from the Sea. The narrow little streets give it its old European appeal. Mulege's abundance of water made this a desirable mission location in the early 1700's. Date, fig, banana, olive and orange production comprises most of the local livelihood, along with fishing and tourism. It has most of the amenities that you will need, not to mention tasty little restaurants and hotels. Weather conditions along the coast from Mulege to Loreto are typically subtropical. Annual rainfall is about 4 inches (10 cm). The winters can get cool, the summers hot and humid. The **Sierra de Guadalupe** contains the largest number of known prehistoric cave paintings in Baja. Several of the hotels in Mulege can arrange excursions to the more accessible sites.

**Getting There:**  Following Highway 1 will take you into Mulege. An airstrip for private aircraft is located 2 ½ miles (4 km) east of town, next to the Hotel Serenidad.

**Accommodations:**   Mulege has a number of small hotels in and outside of town. The **Casa Granada Bed and Breakfast** is located right next to the river! The **Hotel Vista Hermosa** has a river view, with a restaurant and bar. In town, the **Hotel Las Casitas** is popular and close to everything. It has modest accommodations with a restaurant and bar. The **Hacienda Hotel** is also located in town by town square. The **Hotel Mulege** sits right at the entrance of town and is quite simple. The **Cuesta Del Mar Hotel** is south of town between the highway and Mulege river and just north of town is the **Hotel Punta Palmar.** East of town is Mulege's largest hotel, the **Hotel Serenidad**, which has a restaurant, bar and pool. It is quite popular. The turnoff is 2.1 miles (3.4 km) south of the Mulege bridge on Highway 1.

**Camping:** There are several nice camping areas with river views. The **Huerta Saucedo** is east of town on the south side of the river about a half mile (.8 km) off the highway. There are tent sites and full hookups. Also along the river in the same area is **Jorge del Rio**. The **Eco Mundo Camp** has palapa and tent camping, restaurant and bar. **The Oasis Rio** has full hookups and is east of the Orchard RV Park on the south side of the river. There is also **Poncho's** which has basic camping and all of the camps are well kept.

**Launch Ramps:** All of the ramps are located on the river, so be sure to check the tides when launching and returning as the river can get very shallow in spots. **Villa Maria Isabel RV Park** is located 1.4 miles (2 ¼ km) south of the Rio Santa Rosalia bridge. It has a 12 ft. (3.6m) wide ramp composed of a concrete and rock mix. The **Lighthouse ramp** is along the north bank of the river towards the lighthouse 2.5 miles (4 km) and is made of hard packed sand and small rocks. The slope is adequate to handle most boats. The **Orchard ramp** surface is rough concrete and 12 ft. (3.6m) wide and is located .7 miles (1.1 km) past the Rio Santa Rosalia bridge on Highway 1. Turn left at the RV park sign. This ramp is not usable, nor is the river navigable at low tide. Check in at the park office before launching.

***(Punta Chivato)***   Punta Chivato is part of the surrounding area of Mulege. South of the town of Santa Rosalia and north of the town of Mulege on Highway 1, there is a turnoff which takes you several miles on a road leading to Punta Chivato. There you'll find the very beautiful hotel **Posada de las Flores'** which overlooks the Sea of Cortez. There is a small community that resides here. There is a launch ramp, a small store for supplies and water and also an airstrip for small planes. As far as **camping**, there is beach camping with no amenities. But there are also palapas which have restrooms nearby. A new park with hookups is on the drawing board.

## Diving Facilities:
**Cortez Explorers** is a full service dive shop, equipped with scuba & snorkeling equipment, boats and a compressor. They are located on the main street in Mulege. They take day trips to the Santa Inez Islands and Pt. Concepcion.

## Diving & Snorkeling:
The areas surrounding Mulege consist of the northernmost **Isla Tortuga**, which is quite a distance out to sea from Santa Rosalia; **Isla San Marcos** off Punta Chivato; **Isla Santa Inez**, which is a small group of three islands a few miles further south; islands in the **Bahia de Concepcion**, **Punta Concepcion**; and **Isla San Ildefonso** which is over 25 miles (40 km) to the south. The majority of the area has low-lying reefs made up of angular boulders and rock formations. There are large populations of reef fishes, rays, invertebrates, shellfish and along the outer rocky points, sea lions. Like many of Baja's offshore islands, they appear to be lonely, desolate outposts, yet beneath its deceiving appearance, the underwater landscape and marine life are in sharp contrast to the land above the water.

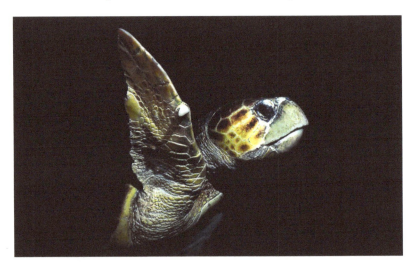

**The loggerhead turtle live most of their life in openwater and spend time on the ocean floor. The shore waters are their main foraging habitat.**

### BLUE WATER DIVING
By swimming out into blue water from deep-water pinnacles or seamounts, divers can often see large pelagic animals that are rarely seen on the shallow reefs; such as tuna, swordfish, marlin, sailfish, hammerhead sharks, schools of large jacks, barracuda and jellyfishes. The best way to blue water dive is to have the panga driver follow your bubbles in case the current picks up. Diving the blue water at about 60ft (18m) can give divers that 'Alice in Wonderland' feeling which can be disorienting. Remember, your buddy is a good reference point and bubbles always float up. Be sure to keep an eye on your depth gauge as it is easy to drop deeper than you plan.

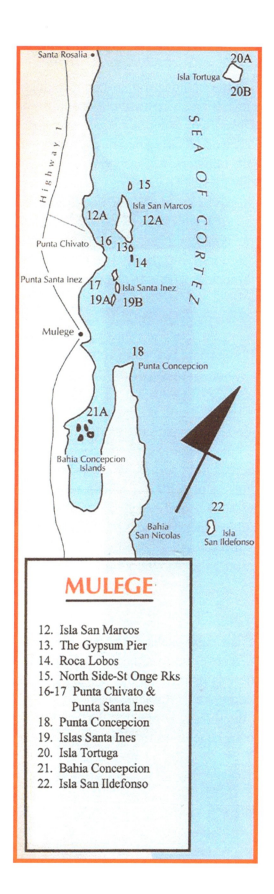

## MULEGE

12. Isla San Marcos
13. The Gypsum Pier
14. Roca Lobos
15. North Side-St Onge Rks
16-17  Punta Chivato &
          Punta Santa Ines
18. Punta Concepcion
19. Islas Santa Ines
20. Isla Tortuga
21. Bahia Concepcion
22. Isla San Ildefonso

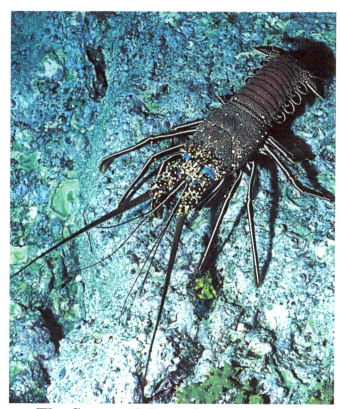

**The Socorro lobster forages around
at night in search of food.**

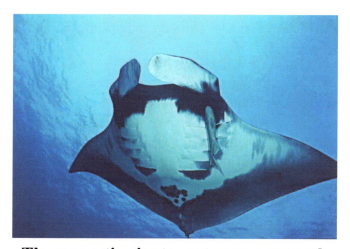

**The magestic giant manta ray can reach
a wingspan of over 18ft (6m) across.**

## 12.  ISLA SAN MARCOS

**THE DEPTH** circumventing San Marcos island ranges from about 20-60+ ft (6-18+m). The island is 5 ½ miles (9 km) long and 2 miles (3.2 km) wide and sits 5 miles (8 km) north of the hotel at Punta Chivato and a mile (1.6 km) offshore.

The underwater terrain on the **East and West Sides (12A)** of the island is similar in appearance. They are dominated by big scattered boulders and rocky outcroppings. Beginning in about 20ft (6m) of water, the boulders spill down a gradual slope into deeper water. Divers will encounter small drop-offs, ledges and deep cavities. Reef fishes are in abundance on both sides. The odd looking bumphead parrotfish and bright green and orange azure parrotfish can be found among the boulders passageways.

Crevices and holes are home to the large green moray eel, along with striped zebra morays and jewel morays which are dressed in chains of gold spots ringed by dark brown halos. Black durgons cruise the reef with convict tangs and damselfishes. The multi-colored giant hawkfish which grows to over 18 inches (46 cm) hover beneath the craggy edges, using its mottled coloration as camouflage.

Invertebrates seem to glide effortlessly over the hard substrate. Red gulf and chocolate chip sea stars feed on algae growth while spiny oysters latch tightly onto coral branches. The entire perimeter of the island is a good area for photography.

## 13.  THE GYPSUM PIER

**THE DEPTH** around and under the pier ranges from 10-40ft (3-12m). There is a small community that lives on San Marcos island which work the gypsum mining operation. The pier where the gypsum is loaded into boats is located on the southwest side of the island and is 290ft (88m) long. The huge, dark pilings frame an incredible underwater setting. Large groupings of reef fish find refuge in this shadowy artificial forest. Schools of cortez chubs, zebra perch, sergeant majors, jacks and cortez angelfish are at times, thick enough to block out much of the sunlight.

**Night Dive:** Night diving on this pier is equally incredible. There is not one inch on the pilings that is not moving with life. Brightly hued anemones are opened up; clusters of golden coral cups are flared out to feed and a variety of purple, gold, blue, white and yellow nudibranchs are everywhere.

The bottom at 40ft (12m) is covered with broken pilings and hunks of metal where critters have found refuge. Octopuses, moray eels, some slipper lobster and an array of invertebrates make their homes here. The large 6 inch (15cm) pink warty sea slug can be found at night under the blanket of pilings. This pier is an excellent spot for close-up and macro photography.

## 14.  ROCA LOBOS

**THE DEPTH** that surrounds Roca Lobos is 18-50ft (6-15m). This particular site is a rock a few hundred yards off the southern tip of Isla San Marcos that rises 20ft (6m) above the sea. The reef and shoals here are very wide and in some places as shallow as 6ft (2m). There is fish life among the jagged reef formations. Shellfish such as tiger paw, scallops and chocolate clams are prominent. Interesting story is, an older local man says that he found pewter plates here in the 1950's while free-diving. Buried wreckage…..who knows? **Caution:** Boats need to be careful when approaching this area because of the many shallow rocks.

## 15.  NORTH SIDE and St. Onge Rocks

**THE DEPTH** here is around 30-80ft (9-24m). This north end of Isla San Marcos offers good diving and snorkeling. Prominent rocky points with numerous detached rock formations characterize the shoreline. Depths start at about 30ft (9m), dropping gradually close to the points. On the northeast side, there is a group of rocks that some call 'St. Onge Rocks' which sit clustered together. Sea lions fill the air with their barking, while in swift silence their brethren barrel underwater around the reef. The rocks are filled with colorful waving gorgonians and sea fans. Grouper, pargo and cabrilla hang out on these offshore rock groupings along with a wide variety of reef fishes.

**Caution:** Currents can become strong in between these rocks. If the surface water shows any rippling pattern, it is best to choose another dive site.

## 16. PUNTA CHIVATO and 17. PUNTA SANTA INES

THE DEPTH at these sites begins at about 5ft (2m) and gradually slopes to about 50ft (15m). These areas can be reached by shore. Approximately 10 miles (16 km) north of Mulege are two points jutting from Baja's mainland. One is **Punta Santa Inez** and the other is **Punta Chivato** which is one mile (1.6 km) to the north. Punta Chivato lies in front of the hotel. The depths here begin very shallow and the bottom is a rock jungle abundant with shellfish and small reef fishes. This is an excellent area for snorkeling.

Punta Santa Inez can be reached by either boat or by dirt road from the hotel at Punta Chivato. The underwater reef system here extends several hundred yards directly offshore. The reef is surrounded by a sandy bottom where depths start at about 10ft (3m) gradually descending to 50ft (15m). Colorful gardens of hard corals, sponges and sea fans dot the reef. Schools of tangs and sergeant majors glide over the maze of rocks while parrotfishes, puffers and triggerfishes are seen solo. Little fish such as the yellow and red striped rainbow wrasse, the checkerboard patterned longnose hawkfish and the largemouth blenny swim slowly among the tops of rocks, only to scurry away in a frantic dash. In the sandy patches, one can find sand anemones, rays, crown of thorn starfish and the huge two-foot (62cm) brown sea cucumbers. During the day lobster are often betrayed by their antennae protruding from under ledges. This is another good area for snorkeling.

## 18. PUNTA CONCEPCION

THE DEPTH surrounding the point at Punta Concepcion is 20-60ft (6-18m). The point sits on the east side of Bahia Concepcion, which is about a 45 minute boat ride from Mulege. The visibility on the point rarely exceeds 50ft (15m) and there are few currents here. At a 20ft (6m) depth there are piles of huge boulders which have formed a wall that drops to a sandy bottom at 60ft (18m).

Large balloonfish can be seen swimming along the edge of the boulders. The sandy area is cobbled with smaller rocks. Spotted tiger snake eels slither over the granulated floor, living in small round holes in the sand which they enter tail first. Look for other holes in the sand floor as the peacock mantis shrimp sits hiding, waiting for a quick meal to pass by. Up to 12 inches (31 cm) long, these colorful little crustaceans are very inquisitive and are quite interesting to observe. They have a sharp razor-like appendage that can cause quite a cut. But carefully wiggling a tidbit close to their hole makes for great photos when their curiosity gets the best of them and they can't resist coming up to peek around. Their eyes will move 360 degrees intently watching you. They usually feed at night on shrimp, snails and small fish.

The large Panamic green morays hide under boulders while fields of garden eels poke their tiny heads above the sandy bottom, quick to disappear as you approach. Triggerfish can be found wedged in narrow crevices and small undercuts are protection to many juvenile fish. Bring your light; you'll be amazed at the little world within the rock formations.

Other areas outside of Bahia Concepcion offer fine beaches, coves and natural harbors ideal for camping and snorkeling. Many rocks and reefs extend seaward from several prominent points and await exploration.

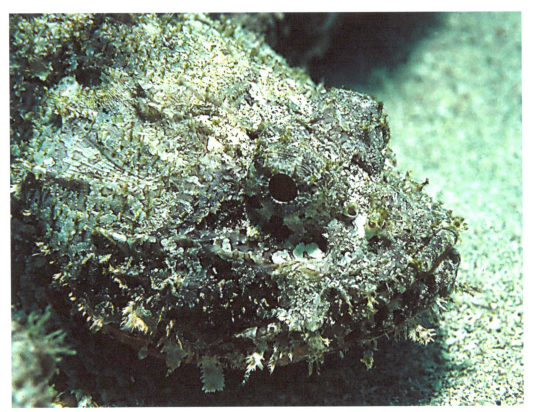

**The scorpionfish is easily camouflaged within the reef.**

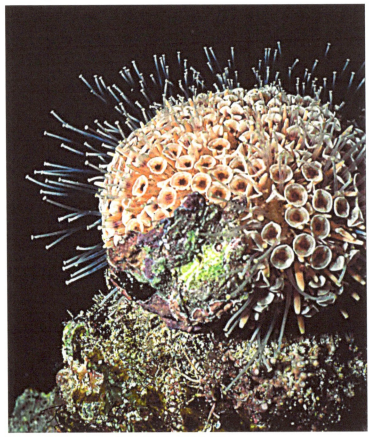

**The flower urchin has the appearance of being covered with tiny pink petals. It likes to cover itself with tiny bits of shells for camouflage.**

## 19. ISLAS SANTA INES

The isles of Santa Ines are a series of three small low-lying islands that are 7 miles (11 km) northeast of Mulege. The southernmost island is the largest, approximately one mile (1.6 km) in length. The other two are somewhat smaller and are separated by shallow patches of submerged rocks.

**The West Side (19A)** which is the leeward side, **THE DEPTH** begins at about 10ft (3m) with a gradual slope to 70ft (21m). They are comprised of a series of sandy alleyways with rocky edges where the bottom levels out to a sandy floor. This is a good area to spot flatfish, rays and halibut. This granular environment is also home to the horse conch. They are still found but not as prolifically as they once were years past. They are the largest native gastropod and can grow up to 18 inches (46 cm) in length. This lovely mollusk has a tan shell and the body of the animal is brilliant red with blue iridescent spots. They make for great photos along with other macro subjects such as a variety of olive snails, nudibranchs and murexes.

**The East Side (19B)** on the seaward side, **THE DEPTH** begins in about 15ft (5m) of water and drops down to over 70ft (21+ m). This side lacks protection from prevailing winds, but sea life is more abundant. The rocky crevices are home to grouper, king and cortez angelfish, cornetfish, trumpetfish and a wide variety of wrasses and damselfishes. In the sandy stretches it is not uncommon to find bullseye stingrays and angel sharks. The visibility fluctuates, but in the late summer and fall months the water is usually clearest. Since there are so many shallow spots around these islands, it is an excellent area for snorkeling as well as scuba diving. The Mexican hogfish, a cousin to the California sheepshead, can be identified by the large hump on the head of the male and two dark stripes on the pink and yellow body of the female. Up to 2 ½ ft (77 cm) long, they are found on the shallow reefs.

## 20. ISLA TORTUGA

Isla Tortuga is a bit of a way out to sea, about 35 miles (56 km) northeast of Mulege and 22 miles (36 km) northeast of Punta Chivato. It is a relatively small island with some small coves. It is not the place you want to be during bad weather. The visibility usually averages between 75-100ft (23-30m).

**The Northeast End (20A)** **also known to some as Pedro Orca**

**THE DEPTH** is 40-100+ ft (12-30+ m). This area has some of the best diving on the island. Here there are layered stair steps of rock and sand. A layer of rock descends for 25ft (8m), then a margin of sand, then another stair step, repeating itself as it plunges into the depths. Amidst the massive boulders, large amounts of leopard grouper can be seen, many weighing over 50 lbs (23 kg). Other fish usually seen here include the panama graysby, spotted cabrilla, red-eyed mutton hamlet, leather bass and a variety of large parrotfishes. Beneath the ledges you can spot the colorful socorro lobster.

**The South End (20B)** **THE DEPTH** ranges from 35-100ft (11-30m). A high sheer cliff on this side of the island drops to the water level, but underwater it is very rocky and not quite as sheer. Car-sized boulders sit delicately balanced upon each other. These monolithic formations create a maze of holes like catacombs. Large panamic green moray eels protrude agape from their lairs. Most of the angelfishes and other reef fishes are much larger here than in other areas, probably because of less human interference. The tiger paw scallops which live in the sand areas average 5-8 inches (13-21 cm) across. They are harvested in enormous quantities by commercial divers. If you're lucky sometimes you can spot a whitetip shark or the exotic looking hammerhead which is always a welcome photo to any photographers collection.

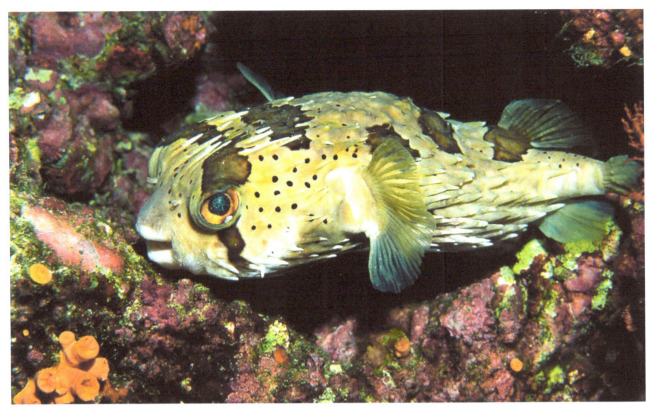

**Covered with spines, the balloonfish puffs up when frightened. It feeds on mollusks and crabs.**

## 21.  BAHIA CONCEPCION

The Bay of Concepcion (Bahia Concepcion) runs north and south and is over 22 miles (36 km) in length. Open to the north and sheltered on the east, the bay has a string of sandy beaches along its west side. **Playa Santispac** has restrooms, showers and large umbrella-like huts with palm-thatched roofs and open sides for camping. Following the unpaved road which parallels the highway provides access to other beaches and campsites.

**Islands of the Bay (21A)** The islands in the Bay of Concepcion have a **DEPTH** beginning at 10ft (3m) and slowly decline to over 60ft (18m). There are half a dozen or so small islands. A couple of them lie within swimming distance from shore, but most are only accessible by boat. Winds can kick up in the afternoons so it's best to plan your dives in the morning. The water around the islands is relatively shallow and is good for snorkeling. In some areas the bottom slopes very gradually eventually reaching a maximum depth of 120ft (36m). The bay is noted for its abundance of pink and black murex shells. Also to be found are colorful sponges, anemones, sea stars, nudibranchs and reef fishes. Shellfish include rock scallops, pen shells, spiny oysters and other mollusks which thrive along the sandy bottom. The visibility is usually fairly limited in the bay, but more than adequate to enjoy snorkeling or diving.

## 22. ISLA SAN ILDEFONSO

**THE DEPTH** around the island of San Ildefonso is 30-100+ ft (9-30+ m). This island is located between Mulege and Loreto, approximately 25 miles (40 km) south of Punta Concepcion by sea and 9 miles (15 km) offshore from San Nicolas Bay. This low-lying island is 1 ½ miles (2.4 km) long and is quite barren. It is surrounded by a steep rocky shoreline. The jagged lava cliffs are inhabited by a menagerie of bird life. There is a large reef 150 yards (136m) off the **southwest point** and the depth drops quickly. Some hammerhead sharks have been seen cruising through in the deeper depths. Few turtles, schools of barberfishes, king angels and surgeonfishes gracefully weave their way through the rocky passageways. These big rock formations and steep pinnacles frame the island, dropping quickly to depths of over 100ft (30m).

On the **west side** of the island there is a large sea lion colony which always makes for a wonderful dive. On the **north end** there is a cluster of offshore rocks and a reef. The radiant colors of the moorish idols, rainbow wrasses, butterflyfishes and the redtail triggerfish which is seldom-seen this far north, create a world of color. Larger fishes such as grouper, snapper, bonito and jacks are likely to be seen here. The island of San Ildefonso is still largely unexplored by scuba divers.

**Caution:** Heavy currents can pick up around this entire area. It is for experienced divers.

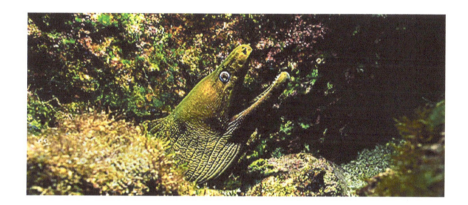

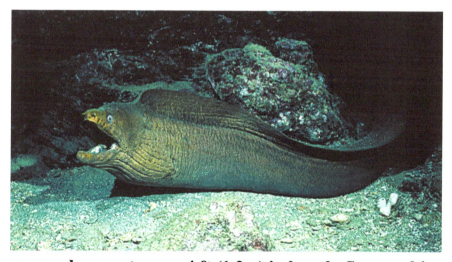

**The green moray eel grows to over 4 ft (1.2m) in length. Seen peeking their heads out from holes during the day, at night they cruise the reef in search of small fish and crustaceans.**

# Chapter VII    LORETO

A Baja reality reminder... 'We still do not know one-thousandth of one percent of what nature has revealed to us'
(Albert Einstein)

**About The Area:**   This town with a population of over 10,000 and growing, was once the first European settlement in the California's and served as the capital for 132 years for a territory that extended as far north as San Francisco. After a hurricane in 1829, Loreto all but vanished for three quarters of a century. Since the completion of Highway 1, Loreto is being discovered by vacationers, sport fishermen, divers and snorkelers. They are drawn to the quiet beauty of this serene area. It is part of the 17 mile (27 km) coast that includes Nopolo and Puerto Escondido.

With a panoramic view of incredible angular, jutting mountain peaks of the Sierra Giganta mountain range which surrounds the area, Loreto and its adjoining communities lay nestled along this island-studded, aqua-blue coastline. Today, Loreto is growing and is becoming one of the number one desired locations for vacationers and divers. This is probably because it has kept its 'old Mexico' charm and has not become the busy, hustle-bustle towns like La Paz and Cabo San Lucas.

**Getting There:**   There are direct daily flights from Los Angeles, San Diego and Tijuana. The airlines that fly to Loreto are; Alaska, Aero California and Aero Mexico. Also following Highway 1 will take you to Loreto if traveling by vehicle.

**Accommodations:**   There are many good hotels to stay at in Loreto. In the center of town by town square is the upscale beautiful **Posada de las Flores**, decorated in an antique Spanish setting. The rooms and restaurant are lovely as is its glass bottom pool. The **La Pinta** is located at the north end of town on the beach. It has nice big rooms w/patio, satellite TV, pool and restaurant/bar. Along the malecon (boardwalk) is the **Oasis**, which has comfortable rooms, pool and restaurant. Also on the malecon is the **Quinta San Francisco** which has simple but clean nice rooms. The **Coco Cabanas** is quite nice, with pool in a quiet setting tucked away down a side street in town. The **Iguana Inn** is another choice with simple clean rooms located on Benito Juarez as well as the quaint and unique **Hotel Luna** located next door to **Dolphin Dive Center**. Off the towns main street is the **Plaza Loreto** and **El Dorado**. Both have restaurant/bar and TV. Close to the highway, just inside town is the **Hacienda Suites**. It is quite nice and has a restaurant/bar and pool. Nopolo, which is 4 miles (6.5 km) south of Loreto is a small, but growing community. There is a higher rating large hotel there. Located on the beach, the **Inn at Loreto Bay** has nice restaurants and pool. About a half hour drive further south, nestled up on a hill with a spectacular view is the **Danzante Private Resort** at Playa Blanca, which is an all-inclusive eco-resort.

**Camping:**   One mile (1.6 km) south of Loreto via Calle Madero is the **Loremar RV Park**. It has full hookups, tent sites, showers, laundry service and thatched roof huts. There is also the **Las Palma RV Park** and **Loreto Shores**. Further south about 15 miles is a trailer park at **Tripui** where a small community resides. Much of the desolate beach areas are still open for camping but have no amenities.

**Launch Ramps:**   From town in Loreto, turn left on the malecon; go .3 miles (.5 km) which takes you to the marina and the **malecon ramp**. The most commonly used 28ft (8.5m) wide ramp is concrete and has good traction. The **Las Palmas RV Park** has a 16ft (4.8m) wide ramp with a concrete rock surface. In town stay to the right of the traffic circle, pass the gas station and continue .6 miles (1 km). Turn right on the dirt road with the RV sign and go .7 miles (1.1 km). The **Marina de Puerto Loreto** is located in Puerto Escondido. Approximately 15 miles (24 km) south of Loreto, turn left at the sign for Tripui RV Park. Go 1.4 miles (2.3 km) and turn into the parking lot. The ramp is 33ft (10m) wide, made of concrete and has good traction. There is a fee to launch.

**Diving Facilities:** Conveniently located, **Dolphin Dive Center** is in town on Benito Juarez Ave, ½ block from the malecon and marina. It is a full-service PADI facility equipped with a gear storage drying room and rinse basin for dive gear and cameras. They offer boat trips, rentals, airfills and dive packages. The yummy little restaurant **'Giggling Dolphin'** beside them is open early for diver's convenience. **Las Parras Tours** and **Cormorant Dive Center** are both located in town on the main street. They also offer boat trips, rentals and airfills as does **Baja Outpost**, which is located on the Malecon. The **Danzante Resort** is a very nice ecological resort located 25 miles south of Loreto. Also **Empresas Rojo** located off Benito Juarez is a good place to purchase marine hardware.

**Diving and Snorkeling:** There are five islands that sit offshore from Loreto. All five are now part of the protected underwater park and marine sanctuary. **Isla Coronado** is 1 ½ miles (2.4 km) offshore and 6 miles (10 km) north of Loreto. **Isla Carmen** is 8 miles (13 km) east of Loreto. **Isla Danzante** is approximately 14 miles (23 km) south of Loreto and a few miles offshore from Puerto Escondido. Further offshore is **Isla Monserrate** and even further, **Isla Catalina**. These islands offer quite diversity, including shallow rocky bottoms, walls with deep canyons, a couple of wreck sites and many reef systems. All are teeming with colorful marine life. There are several pristine white sand beaches along their shores where one can relax. Water clarity usually ranges from 50-100ft (15-30m). The summer and fall months bring in warmer water, around 80+ degrees F (27+ C). Besides the local species of tropical fishes, seasonal game fish frequent these waters, the most common being jacks, dorado, yellowtail, roosterfish and snapper. In early summer and fall large Humboldt squid pass through the channel, as they migrate to shallower waters to lay their eggs and mate.

Many whales and dolphins also pass through these channels. It is not uncommon to see and sometimes even snorkel with pods of pilot whales and schools of dolphins. The winter months bring in the massive blue whales, humpbacks and some grays. During the winter and spring the water cools down to where a 7mm wetsuit is recommended.

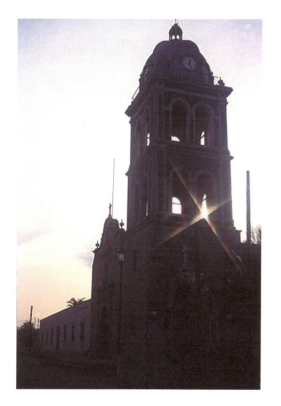

**The 'Mision Nuestra Senora De Loreto' is one of Loretos historical landmarks. The first building of this mission began in 1699. The floor was laid in 1704 and the church was completed by 1752. Beside the church is an interesting museum.**

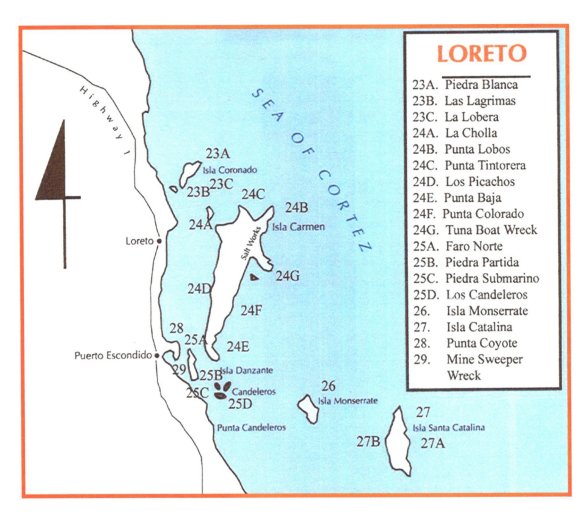

### LORETO

23A. Piedra Blanca
23B. Las Lagrimas
23C. La Lobera
24A. La Cholla
24B. Punta Lobos
24C. Punta Tintorera
24D. Los Picachos
24E. Punta Baja
24F. Punta Colorado
24G. Tuna Boat Wreck
25A. Faro Norte
25B. Piedra Partida
25C. Piedra Submarino
25D. Los Candeleros
26.   Isla Monserrate
27.   Isla Catalina
28.   Punta Coyote
29.   Mine Sweeper
       Wreck

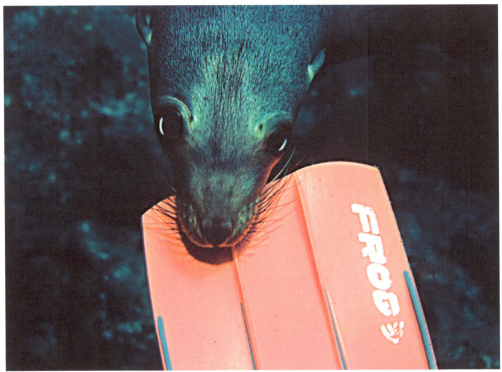

**A friendly sea lion promotes a diver to play.**

## 23. ISLA CORONADO

Looking as if some giant played a hand in molding this island from clay, its awesome appearing majestic pillars and steeples are made of huge volcanic rocks. Coronado island has many very good dive sites.

**Piedra Blanca (23A) THE DEPTH** ranges from 35-100+ ft (11-30+ m). This northeast side is a very interesting site. The currents can pick up so it usually becomes a drift dive. Massive boulders appear to have toppled like dominoes down the declining wall. The underwater terrain is as exquisitely sculptured as the formations on the island itself. At 60ft (18m) a steep drop-off starts, continuing down into the depths. This wall is fractured with deep slices and wide fissures, along with drooping overhangs. Purple gorgonian sea fans sporadically dot the wall. Clumps of golden black coral bushes can be seen as shallow as 60ft (18m) but grow more profusely in deeper water where at 150ft (45m) the bottom is covered. Rock scallops are scattered in clumps across the ledges along with a variety of invertebrates. Schools of triggerfish are plentiful at this end, as are the bumphead parrotfish. Divers can find a variety of pufferfish, such as the bullseye puffer, the polka dotted guineafowl puffer, the balloonfish and the huge spotted porcupinefish that grows to 3ft (0.9m) in length, hovering within rocky channels or resting on the sandy channel bottoms. This entire drift dive offers a great variety of marine life and unusual looking terrain.

**Las Lagrimas (23B) THE DEPTH** starts at around 20ft (6m), dropping down to 80ft (24m). Located at the south end of the island, this area is made up of rocky outcroppings. A jumble of good sized boulders creates a refuge for fishes and moray eels. There is usually a slight current, so pangas follow the divers. Southwest of the point, a reef extends out to where monolithic rocks overlap each other down a gradual slope. There are small grottos throughout the rocks which harbor octopuses, some lobster and many reef fishes such as the Mexican hogfish, hawkfish, damselfish and angelfish.

On the east side near the south end is a very nice cove for snorkeling. The shallow bottom is a great spot to find chocolate clams just beneath the sand. Also look down into the holes that you find in the sand. Many are homes to the finespotted jawfish, where it makes the walls of the hole out of little rocks and shells, 'very artistic'. They have a very wide mouth where they incubate their eggs. As they poke their little heads up to look around for small bottom dwelling animals to feed on, it is an ideal time to snap a photo or simply just observe them.

**La Lobera (23C) THE DEPTH** ranges from 20-100ft (6-30m). This is a beautiful dive. Beginning shallow, you follow the rocks around the point to a colorful wall that drops down to 100ft+. The wall is filled with waving sea fans, sponges, invertebrate life and an array of reef fishes. A sea lion colony lives just above on the island so these inquisitively playful guys will zoom past, only to stop at times to pose for a photo. Once around the point, you will come up to the top plateau. On many occasion divers will see a swirling school "sometimes in the hundreds' of patrolling Mexican barracuda and large fish. The shallower areas of this site are also great for snorkeling.

## 24. ISLA CARMEN

Isla Carmen is one of the largest islands in the Sea of Cortez. It is over 18 miles (29 km) in length and once had a large salt mining operation. It sits 8 miles (13 km) east of Loreto and is surrounded by protected bays and coves. There are many very good diving and snorkeling areas around the points and protruding rock formations. The island is characterized by steep rocky bluffs with a number of large detached rocks around the points.

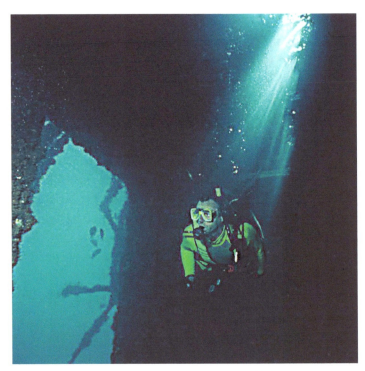

**A diver explores the tuna boat wreck off Carmen Is. Loreto.**

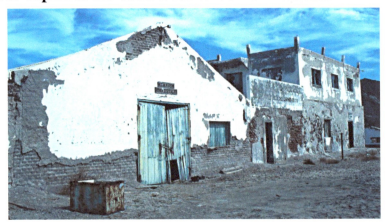

**The abandoned salt works on Carmen Is. Loreto.**

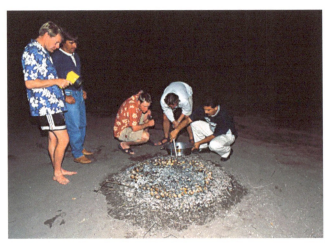

**A Mexican style clambake, using tumbleweeds.**

**La Cholla (24A)** THE DEPTHS range from about 15-60+ ft (5-18+ m). This small detached islet sits north of Carmen island. Depths begin shallow then drop to 60ft (18m) where a sloping rock and sand bottom meander down into deeper water. Diving around this small islet is excellent. There is a great diversity of marine life. Colorful tropical fish inhabit the area and in spring and early summer there is an abundance of juveniles. The brightly colored iridescent yellow and sky blue markings of the juvenile cortez angelfish and the brilliant gold and blue lines of the juvenile king angel make for incredible photos. And don't forget to look between the rock slivers as you may spot the master of disguise, the ever enchanting, octopus.

**Punta Lobos (24B)** THE DEPTHS range from 20-60ft (6-18m) and this site is located at the far north tip of the island. This area usually has good diving whether the winds are coming from the southeast or northwest. When it is too rough on one side of the point, you can often dive the other side, although there can be some surge. The shallow areas are good for snorkeling and divers can work their way down to an intermediate slope to 60ft (18m) with a gradual slope that extends deeper.

This area is excellent for seeing large grouper, bass and parrotfish. It is sometimes difficult to see the mottled scorpionfish that lie motionless around the rocks, but sudden movement quickly jolts their instincts to move. They are great subjects for photographers because they are easy to approach, but because of their poisonous dorsal spines they should not be approached too closely. Some divers call this spot moray city because divers can see moray eels in and around all the grottos and fissures. At around 40-50ft (12-15m) hard coral is growing.

**Punta Tintorera (24C)** THE DEPTHS here begins as shallow as 15ft (5m), dropping down to 60+ ft (18+ m). Located on the northwest side of the island, gigantic boulders make up the shallow reef while smaller rocks are nestled on the bottom at depths beyond 60ft (18m). Throughout this rocky reef are chiseled passageways of sand and coralline algae. Along the tops of and in cavities cut in the rocks, look for patches of purple. Swimming back and forth over them will be a sergeant major. The purple patches are their eggs. Oddly enough, it is the male fish that guards the nest from predators. Goatfish and triggerfish are seen in abundance. All sizes of moray eels can be found spotted moving about beneath the protruding shelves. On the sandy floor there will be what looks like little craters in the sand. These are the nests of triggerfish where they fan out a hole with their fins, then lay eggs. At certain times of the year they will perform quite a dance ritual over these craters, warning all, to stay away.

**Los Picachos (24D)** THE DEPTHS range from 15-100ft (5-30m). Located further south on Carmen's western shoreline, you will come to some fantastic lava cliffs. Caves have been carved into the cliffs by eons of wind and water action. Sun-dappled reflections from the water flicker and dance on the cave walls. The massive cliffs continue down underwater almost vertically to about 100ft (30m). The walls are sprinkled with red and purple gorgonians, as well as yellow and brown sea fans. Grouper, pargo and scrawled filefish, along with an array of other marine critters can be found around the sculpted crevices. Diving conditions are almost always good due to protection from southerly winds.

**Punta Baja (24E)** THE DEPTHS range from 15-50ft (5-15m). This site is located at the southern tip of Isla Carmen. The sea floor stays relatively shallow for a distance from shore. The granite rocks are filled with cracks and cubby holes. The water is usually quite clear as there is not much sediment and it is filled with a diverse variety of marine life. Don't overlook the seemingly barren sand bottom. Particularly interesting to watch is the Pacific razorfish, a little wrasse about 10 inches (26cm) long. When approached, it will actually dart head first into the sand, totally disappearing. Because of their razor-like profiles and compressed bodies, they can swim laterally under the sand when threatened. Identified by two very long spines of the first dorsal fin, giving a 'unicorn' appearance and distinctive body shape distinguish this wrasse from others in the Gulf of California. Several species of flatfish, including halibut, linger in the sand mounds along with the cortez round stingray, bullseye stingray and the bullseye electric ray, which can give you a bit of a jolt. Invertebrates such as the flower urchin 'which is covered with what looks like little pink petals', colorful sand anemones and the feathery sea pen are common here.

**Caution:** Currents can pick up and sweep around the point, so exercise caution.

**Punta Colorado (24F)** **THE DEPTHS** range from 35-60+ ft (11-18+ m). This point is on the east side towards the south end of Isla Carmen. At an average depth of 35ft (11m) is a reef system which runs parallel to the shoreline. Of volcanic origin, the reef is full of short crevices. Lobster can be found in the rock cavities along with a variety of other reef dwellers. Varieties of very colorful gobys make for great photos. These little fish have an almost cartoon looking face as do their very similar buddies, the blennies. This shallow area is also an excellent spot for snorkeling.

**Tuna Boat Wreck (24G)** **THE DEPTH** at this wreck site is 35ft (11m). On the east side towards the north of Isla Carmen is a large bay named Bahia Salina. This is where the salt-making operation used to be and you can still see the large salt pond beyond the bay. In 1985, the small town of Bahia Salina was abandoned when salt-making ceased to be profitable. Much of the old buildings still stand. Doors squeak open and close, then slam in the wind. Salt carts are silent on their tracks beside the remains of a rusty beached shipwreck. But the most interesting is the little church that is still intact. From the gold-leafed Madonna still set behind glass to the nativity set standing on a table, it is almost as if the little church is just waiting for its congregation to return.

As interesting as this little community is, the highlight for divers lies about a half mile (.8 km) outside the bay. Here the remains of a 120ft (36m) Mexican fishing boat, once part of the Ensenada tuna fleet, poke above the water. The ship went down in 1981 when a butane tank blew up, and the ship caught fire and sank. She now lies in 35ft (11m) of water on her port side. The stability of the wreck is questionable, so be wary of penetrating it.

For photography, however, this wreck is sensational. On a bright day, sunlight streaks through the openings of the wreckage, exposing parts inside. Thousands of fish linger about its skeletal frame. Schools of barracuda, angelfishes, snapper, trumpetfish, grunts and jacks move through the sunlight like glittery sheets. The visibility is only about 30ft (9m) as the wreckage sits on a silt sand bottom which gets kicked up by currents and surge. There are parts of the wreck that even have some golden black coral bushes growing on it. The glass windows are still intact, but radio gear and other bits of wreckage lie strewn across the sandy floor.

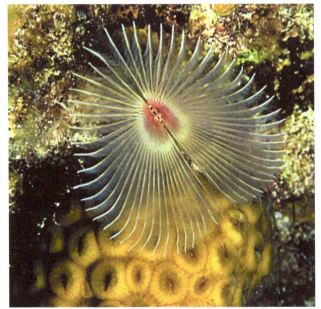

**A Fanworm opens to feed. Living in membranous tubes, they can withdraw quickly when disturbed. They are approximately 1-2 in. (25-50mm)**

## GENTLE GIANTS · THE GRAY WHALES OF BAJA

Each year, from January through March, an estimated 17,000 Pacific gray whales mate and give birth in Baja's Pacific lagoons and some areas in the Sea of Cortez. Their yearly migration from Alaska's Bering Sea is one of the longest on record for any mammal. Once spring arrives, they will head back north again swimming at 4—5 knots paralleling the coastline for about 5000 miles (8065 km) each way, feeding on krill, pelagic red crabs and eelgrass. They reach lengths of 50ft (15m) long and weigh 40 tons (36mt).

At birth, calves measure nearly 15ft (5m) and weigh almost a ton (1.1mt). Their growth is rapid, sustained by a thick 55% milk fat. They are known for their high intelligence and tender demeanor among other whales and humans. During mating, their slow courtship of touching often involves two males and one female. Gestation period is about a year. Baby calves swim by their mothers, watching and repeating all her actions. When the mother stops to rest, the playful baby will cross back and forth over her, pulling itself on her back and tease her until she plays. These whales are friendly and enjoy human contact, rolling over to have their tummy's and head scratched. It is an amazing experience to have one of these magnificent creatures nuzzling against you. Once hunted and slaughtered to almost extinction, the gray whale has made a remarkable comeback and in January 1993 it was taken off the endangered list. The lagoons are now official sanctuaries and no boats are permitted in certain lagoons. 'Charles Scammon', a whale hunter at the turn of the century, states that 'after slaughtering one of the mother whales, she was tied to the side of the ship and her young calf followed the ship swimming beside her dead body for over two days until it had no more strength to go on.' He also states that many of the motherless calves huddled together in a small circle, confused and frightened... Preventing future atrocities such as these lie solely in our hands. The protection of whales, marine life and all animals on this planet is our sole responsibility.    Think........

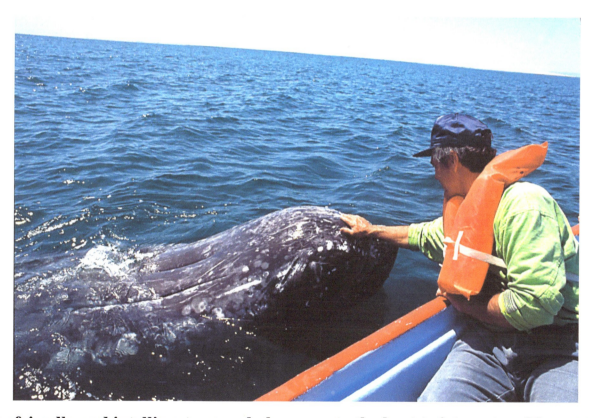

**The friendly and intelligent gray whales come to the boat to interact and be petted.**

## 25. ISLA DANZANTE

This small island is located off the southwest side of Isla Carmen, 2 ½ miles (4 km) offshore of Puerto Escondido. The shore on the north end of the island is characterized by steep rocky points. This is a beautiful island to explore and hike around on.

**Faro Norte (25A)** **THE DEPTHS** range from 15-100+ ft (5-30+ m). Faro Norte is located on the northeast side of Isla Danzante. The underwater terrain is a series of short walls that eventually drop to over 100ft (30m). There are deep canyons and crevices lined with hard and soft corals, and below the 50ft (15m) depth are a lot of black coral bushes. The short walls are made up of heavy block-like boulders which make wonderful homes for marine life. Local reef fishes can be found throughout the area and octopuses are often seen here.

**Piedra Partida (25B)** **THE DEPTHS** range from around 15-60+ ft (5-18+ m). This site is located on the east side of Isla Danzante. There are a number of places on this side to dive. Shallow diving around 20ft (6m) is interesting as there is a wide variety of reef fishes swimming throughout the rocky terrain. The white sandy areas seem to attract an ample number of parrotfishes. There is usually a current here, so this is often a drift dive at around 60ft (18m) while the pangas follow. The reef which extends off the southeastern point shoots to deeper depths with sheer vertical walls. Use a dive light even in the daytime to really bring out the colors, especially of marine life hidden back in the deep crevices. A light can bring into focus a matrix of life forms.

**Piedra Submarino (25C)** **THE DEPTHS** here range from 15-100ft (5-30m). From a distance El Submarino (submarine rock) has the appearance of a submarine. Located off the south tip of the island, this monolithic structure is made up of short walls with intervening crevices running back into the rocks. The shallow slope extends southwards towards Candeleros. The west side of this giant rock formation drops off quickly. The surrounding area is great for exploring, as the ledges and undercuts provide a habitat for colorful murex snails and other mollusks. Sea stars, such as the purple star, the red gulf star and the chocolate chip star are also found here as are octopuses, rock scallops and few lobsters.

**Los Candeleros (25D)** **THE DEPTHS** here range from 40-80+ ft (12-24+ m). Los Candeleros (the candlesticks) is named for three large rock pinnacles which sit between the south tip of Isla Danzante and Punta Candeleros on Baja's mainland. Sitting several hundred yards from each other, these pinnacles are visible from Puerto Escondido. They look like gigantic granite steeples, rising from the depths. The peak on the north side is called **Islotes Colorado** and is so loaded with sea stars that the water sometimes has an odor of iodine, a chemical they release. The second pinnacle is called **Islotes Tijeras**, referring to the scissor tail of the prehistoric-looking frigate bird. This area is part of their nesting grounds. The third pinnacle is known as **Islotes Pardo**, referring to its dark color and plunging depths.

The shallower areas around the pinnacles are made up of short walls and clumps of rocks. Numerous submerged large boulders lie close to the shore while larger jutting boulders loom upwards from the depths. Marine life is prolific around these submarine cathedrals. The drop-offs and drooping ledges are also quite dramatic and make for excellent photographs.

The middle pinnacle is connected to a smaller rock formation off the northwest side by a shallow channel. This spot is good for snorkeling. Large game fishes, including grouper and yellowtail are common around the pinnacles especially in deeper water. The Candeleros are really recommended for those with deep water experience.

## 26. ISLA MONSERRATE

The island of Isla Monserrate is located 8 miles (13 km) from Baja's nearest mainland point. The island is a low-lying volcanic land mass that appears barren. It is 4 miles (6.5 km) long and 2 miles (3.2 km) wide. Around the shoreline the depths are shallow, but drop quickly to deeper water. The southeast side forms a series of finger-like reefs. Sandy narrow channels intrude throughout the reef-fingers. Marine life around Monserrate is typical of that found throughout the Loreto area. This island along with Isla Catalina is quite remote and not frequently dived. They are great areas for those coming to Baja with their own long range boat. But for those that do not have a boat and are interested in diving these outer islands, possible trips can be arranged through a local dive shop. Two miles north of Monserrate are some small islets called **La Reinita** that offers great diving. Pinnacle walls, and rocky ledges make up the structure. Fish are more readily seen here in larger schools.

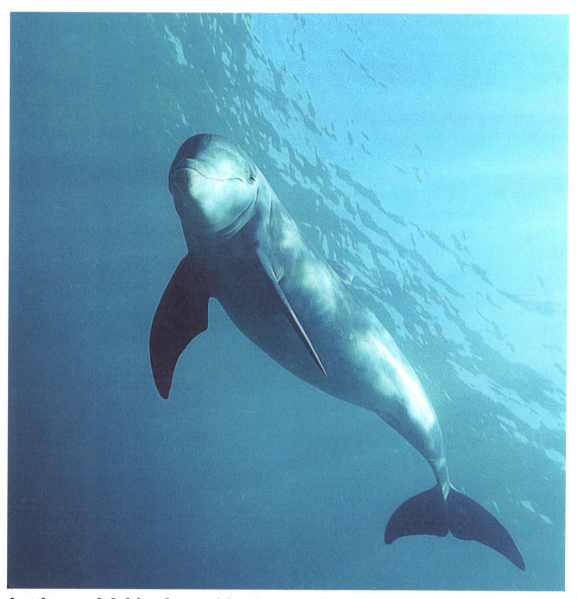

**The bottlenose dolphin along with other species of dolphins thrive throughout the Sea of Cortez.**

## 27.  ISLA CATALINA

Isla Catalina is quite remote, sitting 12 miles (19 km) southeast of Isla Monserrate. It is 8 miles (13 km) long and 2 miles (3.3 km) wide.

**East Side (27A)**  THE DEPTHS range from 20-100+ ft (6-30+ m). With an underwater terrain made up of a series of sheer angular cliffs which continue underwater, this is a great area for seeing larger fishes, turtles, occasional manta rays and sharks. But be sure to watch the currents as they can pick up.

**West Side (27B)**  THE DEPTHS also range from about 20-100+ ft (6-30+ m). But the underwater terrain is quite different in appearance. Here, there are more protected coves and beaches nestled in the rocky shoreline. The points which encompass the coves are excellent sites for diving, with depths as shallow as 20ft (6m). Inside the crevices found on the rock canopies, divers will discover scallops and lobster, large populations of reef fishes, invertebrates and rays, along with seasonal schooling mobulas (small type manta rays) and occasional nurse sharks.

## 28.  PUNTA COYOTE

THE DEPTHS range from 15-60+ ft (5-18+ m). From Puerto Escondido off the mainland, divers can have a panga drop them off at Punta Coyote. This point is located northward and outside of the bay. With large rocks and boulders that have tumbled down a gentle slope, the diving is not spectacular, but it is good. Gorgonians and sea fans are sprinkled over the reef below 60ft (18m). These giant boulders are very interesting to explore. Angelfish, pufferfish, butterflyfish and a myriad of tiny fast-swimming wrasses and damselfish inhabit the area. Gulf stars cover the sand bottom and a few types of rays like to hang out here. Also keep an eye out for the cartoon-looking jawfish that peeks its head out from holes. They are wonderful photographic subjects. This is also a great site for a night dive because of its easy accessibility by boat. Darkness brings out the huge, hairy elegant hermit crabs, lobster, free-swimming moray eels, long-legged arrow crabs and few nudibranchs. Brilliantly colored golden cup corals and anemones open up to feed creating a kaleidoscope of color.

## 29.  MINE SWEEPER WRECK

THE DEPTH on the top of the bridge is 35ft (11m) and the bottom sits on the sandy bottom at 75ft (23m). This C-54 Mine Sweeper is 150ft (45m) long. Built and operated by the U.S. Navy, it was decommissioned and sold to Mexico's Navy. The ship was sunk intentionally for a dive site and it sits upright. Usually marked by a float, it is ½ mile (.8 km) offshore in the bay and a short distance south of Puerto Escondido.

This wreck is a wonderful dive. At certain times of the year, it can have  thousands of cortez grunts, hundreds of graysbys and in the open blue around the wreck; you will occasionally see lookdowns, which is an interesting looking fish as it always looks as though it is sadly looking down. Where these fish go during other times of the year is a mystery. Turtles frequent this area as well, sometimes resting on the skeletal frame. The holds and rooms of the wreck are great to explore and make for awesome photos. Streams of sunlight filter through the open areas below while schools of circling fish move in a rhythmic motion that is literally mesmerizing.

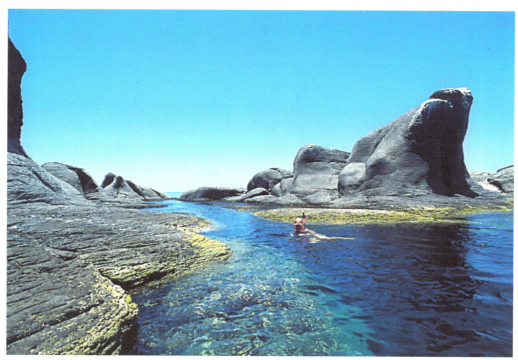
**Some great places to snorkel at Coronado Is. Loreto**

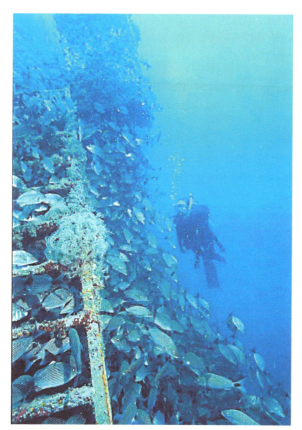
**Resting in 75 ft (23m) of water, the 150 ft (45m) long C-54 mine sweeper wreck is a great dive, off Puerto Escondido.**

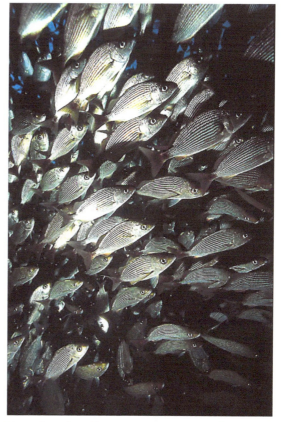
**Hundreds of grunts swarm the mine sweeper wreck.**

# Chapter VIII       LA PAZ

**About The Area:**   La Paz (meaning Peace) now lives up to its name after being one of the most violent towns on the peninsula in previous centuries. This was the site of the first Spanish attempt to settle what at that time was believed to be an island called Santa Cruz. The captain of the expedition, Diego Becerra, was murdered by his crew in 1533. Shortly after, the new leader, Fortun Jimenez and twenty two of his soldiers were killed by the Indians. Spain's most infamous conquistador, Hernan Cortez, himself, led a group of soldiers and colonists to La Paz. Eventually this group returned to the mainland because of the difficulty of replenishing supplies.

The first permanent colony was formed in 1811. In 1829 following the big hurricane that damaged Loreto, La Paz was named the capital of the Southern Territory of California. The prime lure of La Paz was the rich pearl oyster beds. In the 18th century, many of the finest pearls of the royal treasury in Spain came from La Paz. Pearling continued until the 1940's when a mysterious disease destroyed the oyster beds in the Sea of Cortez. The 1950's brought sports fishermen from the U.S. and La Paz acquired the reputation of being one of the bill fishing capitals of the world. It was commonly visited by North American literati and Hollywood celebrities and after the completion of Highway 1 the city became a tourist destination for mainland Mexicans. Statehood was bestowed on the Territory of Baja California Sur in 1974 and La Paz, which has over 100,000 residents, was crowned the capital.

One place worth visiting is the Museum of Anthropology, where exhibits cover the cape region's anthropology from prehistoric to modern times. On display are fossils, minerals, Indian artifacts and maps of rock-painting sites throughout central and southern Baja. There are restaurants for all tastes and budgets in La Paz, many located along the main waterfront.

**Getting There:**   There are daily flights to La Paz. The airlines that fly there are Alaska, Aero California and Aero Mexico. If coming to La Paz by vehicle, just continue south on Highway 1.

**Accommodations:**   There are several good hotels to choose from. The **Los Arcos Hotel** is equipped with all the amenities including TV, pool, restaurant/bar. The **Cabanas de Los Arcos** is also quite nice with that old Mexico ambiance. Both the **Fiesta Inn** and the **Crowne Plaza La Paz** have a pool and health club. The **Seven Crown La Paz** has a pool and hot tub. Both the **La Concha Beach Resort** and the **Club Hotel Cantamar** have a pool, hot tub and water sport activities. The **Best Value Inn** has a kitchen, pool and water sport activities. The **Club El Moro** also has water sports activities. All of these hotels are in the medium price range. Some of the lower end priced hotels include the **Hotel La Perla**, the **Hotel Gardenias**, the **Miramar Hotel** and **Nuevo Pekin Hotel**.

**Camping:**   There is beach camping north of the Pichilingue ferry terminal at **Playa Pichilingue**, **Puerto Balandra**, **Puerto El Tecolote** and **Puerto El Coyote**. It is a good idea to bring in your own supplies. There are also trailer parks on the west side of town off Highway 1. A few other RV parks are **Casa Blanca RV park**, **El Cardon Trailer park** and **La Paz RV park**.

**Launch Ramps:**   When approaching La Paz from the north, you will see a large white dove statue. Keep to the left and you will come to the **Fidepaz ramp** on the left. The concrete ramp is 30ft (9m) wide and has good traction. It is located at the far west end of the La Paz channel down the bay.

The **Marina de La Paz ramp** is 3 miles (4.8 km) past the dove statue. Turn left one block before the second stop light and proceed to the ramp. This ramp is 14ft (4.2m) wide and also of good concrete.

The two concrete **Pichilingue ramps** are 12ft (3.6m) wide. To get there; go 10.9 miles (17.6 km) past the Hotel Los Arcos. One half mile (.8 km) past the ferry terminal turn off the highway and follow the dirt road another half mile (.8 km).

## Diving Facilities:

There are several dive operations in La Paz. **Baja Quest** offers dive trips for both day and overnight island camping. **Baja Expeditions** offers one day dive trips and week long trips on the 80ft (24m) liveaboard the 'Don Jose', which holds 16 divers comfortably. They go to the outer islands and seamounts.

Other dive operations that offer rentals, boat trips and airfills are; **Baja Diving & Service/Club Cantamar**, **Scuba Baja Joe**, the **Cortez Club (in La Concha Hotel)**, **Carey Outdoors**, **Sea & Adventures**, **Tio's Sports** by Melia Hotel, and **Fun Baja** at Marina Palmira. There are other diving services that are located at some of the hotels.

## Diving & Snorkeling:

The diving and snorkeling around La Paz consists of a series of islands, islets and seamounts. None of the islands are really inhabited full time, but there are Mexican fish camps which dot the shorelines of some of the larger islands.

Typically, the undersea terrain is characterized by mammoth pieces of broken granite, jumbled rocks and boulders which form unique-looking structures and winding grottos. Many of the huge reef systems are honeycombed with arches, tunnels and caves. There are steep walls that plummet to sand bottoms and mountain peaks that jut up from the sea floor to within 60ft (18m) of the surface. There is an exciting mixture of deep-water pelagics along with inshore reef animals.

Water temperatures during the winter and early spring months are in the 65-75 degree F (18-24 C) range. During the mid-summer and fall months, temperatures reach a warmer 80-85 degrees F (27-29 C). This period is considered the rainy season, but is also the best time for diving. Occasional hurricanes and tropical storms called chubascos can occur usually from June to October. The islands and dive sites are further out than other areas in the Sea of Cortez.

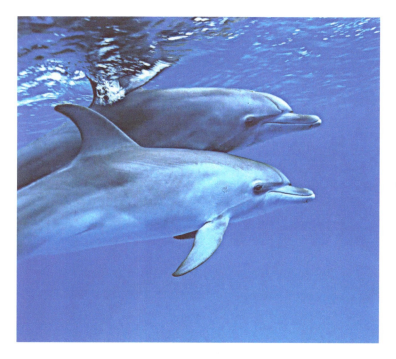

**Most all species of Dolphins will at times, school in the hundreds. They are family oriented and are rarely seen alone.**

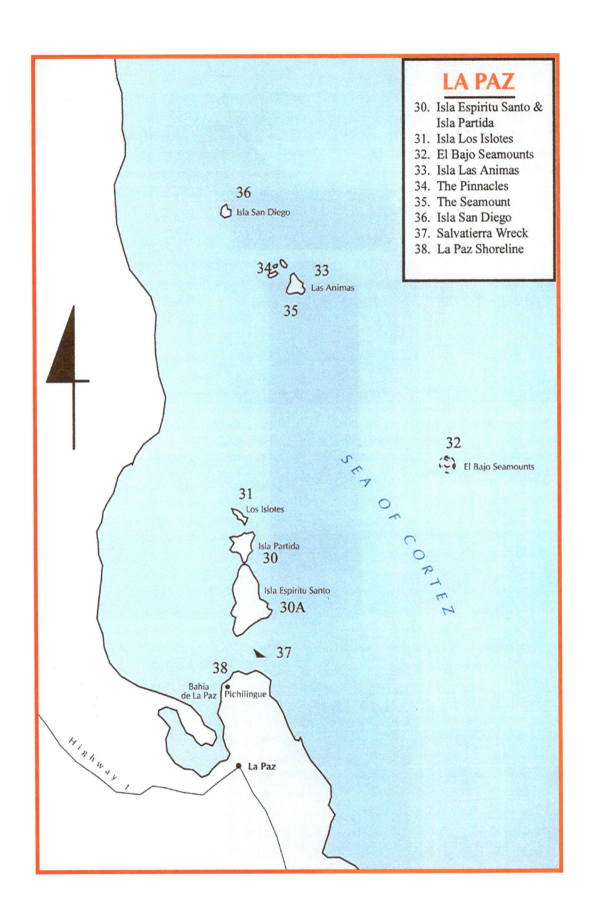

## LA PAZ

36
Isla San Diego

34 33
Las Animas

35

32
El Bajo Seamounts

SEA OF CORTEZ

31
Los Islotes

Isla Partida
30

Isla Espiritu Santo
30A

37

38

Bahia
de La Paz
Pichilingue

Highway 1

La Paz

## 30. ISLA ESPIRITU SANTO and ISLA PARTIDA

**THE DEPTHS** range from 20-100+ ft (6-30+ m) and these islands are located 18 miles (29 km) north of La Paz. Together they are about 15 miles (24 km) in length, with Isla Espiritu Santo being much larger. Isla Partida sits just north of Espiritu Santo and in one small section they are only about 15ft (5m) apart. There are numerous wind-protected coves which line the more protected west sides of both these islands. The rocky reefs around the coves appear barren, but a close inspection will reveal quite a variety of marine life. Snorkeling is good around the west side because of its shallow depths of around 20ft (6m).

Some of the best diving areas are located along the **north end of Isla Partida** and **east side of both islands**, but they are more affected by weather. The rocky points along the east side have a greater variety of marine life and the drop-offs are deeper.

**Punta Lobos (30A)**, which is the most eastern point of Espiritu Santo is a rocky bluff that drops quickly to deep water. Around the point, **DEPTHS** of 80ft (24m) can be easily reached. A 600ft (182m) submarine trench lies about a half mile (.8 km) offshore. The rich nutrients from the deep-water currents provide a constant source of food, which explains the large abundance of marine life. There are over 20 types of commonly-seen, brightly-colored sea stars. The chocolate-chip star looks almost edible. The brilliant pink smooth star and the red cushion star really stand out. Large aggregations of the cushion star are reported in the summer months. Tropicals such as cornetfish, triggerfish, parrotfish, hogfish and grouper are plentiful around the point, so photography can be excellent.

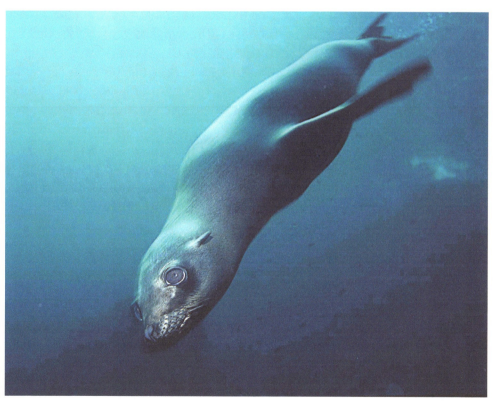

**Sealions are very curious creatures**

## 31. ISLA LOS ISLOTES

**THE DEPTHS** here range from about 25-50ft (8-15m). Located just north of Isla Partida is the small islet of Los Islotes. It is rugged in appearance with awesome-looking angular formations. A tour around the island is a must. California sea lions lie strewn across the sun-dappled rocks, soaking up the warmth. The adolescent sea lions mouth each other in playfulness and courtship. They slide off the rocks, gliding effortlessly through the water. Underwater these furry marine dogs are the clowns of the sea. The lively antics of these big, brown glassy-eyed goofs are overwhelming. Allowing divers to get very close, they will somersault and blow bubbles in your face, only to quickly zip away. Inquisitively, they will gently pull at snorkels and fins. During mating season, the big bulls can become aggressive when they are protecting their harems. They will come at divers head-on, occasionally baring teeth and bellowing a loud bark. For an instant, your vision may be full of bubbles. Remember, like all warnings these should be respected so you should back off. Always, remember, you're the visitor. Easily recognized, these big males are much larger than the females and have a big bump on their heads. Females choose their mate partially on the quality of the shoreline that the male is defending. The males are greatly out-numbered by their harems of females. At about 25ft (8m) there are beautiful undercuts, small caves and grottos. An ecosystem of colorful soft gorgonians and golden cup corals hang in clusters from the grotto ceilings. This islet seems to rate highly in its great diversity of sea stars, each having a kaleidoscope of colors. There are usually large schools of blue and gold king angelfish, yellow surgeonfish and a large variety of other tropicals especially around the east end.

Usually seen in the shallows around 20-25ft (6-8m) deep are massive glittering balls of thousands of anchovies. They move along the reef like great waves of glitter. Once in a while the perfect photo opportunity appears when this glittery ball opens up to let a sea lion through. On the east side of the islet is a huge archway which extends underwater to a depth of 30ft (9m) and goes to the other side of the islet. From past storms, big boulders have shifted into parts of the passageways. But it is an overwhelming sight when schools of fish and sea lions silhouette themselves under this big arch beneath the sun's rays above.

**Great Night Dive:** This arch area also makes for an awesome night dive. The side walls are blanketed with golden cup corals that are open and feeding, guided by their nocturnal time clocks. Guinea puffers have been seen sleeping in crevices along with octopus, turtles and parrotfish. Many of the parrotfish wrap themselves up in a cocoon of mucus which helps protect them from predators by masking their scent. They are easily approached for photos, but be careful; you don't want to disturb them. In the early morning, they will chew their way out of their little sleeping bag, only to abandon it on the reef. You will sometimes see the discarded sleeping attire rolling around in a wad in the surge.

## 32. EL BAJO SEAMOUNTS

**THE DEPTHS** at the seamounts range from 50-100+ ft (15-30+ m). Located east of Isla Espiritu Santo is a group of three submerged pinnacles known as the seamounts. The tops of these mountain peaks begin on the shallowest mount at 50ft (15m) below the surface, dropping to well over 100ft (30m). Manta rays were once abundant here, but due to over-fishing they are less readily seen. Still, occasionally they are sighted gliding over the seamounts. Because of the rich upwelling water from the surrounding depths, this area is a prime location for large pelagic animals. Bigger schools of fish and turtles are common around the seamounts.

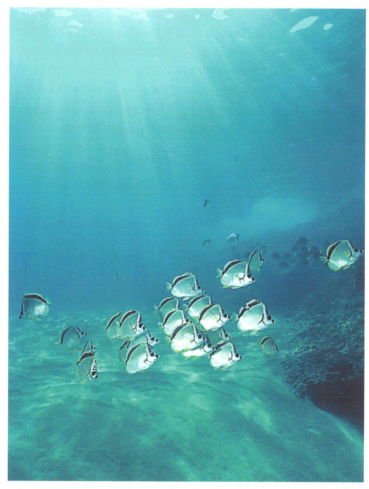

Schools of barberfish can be found around shallow reefs
and also hovering over the sand.

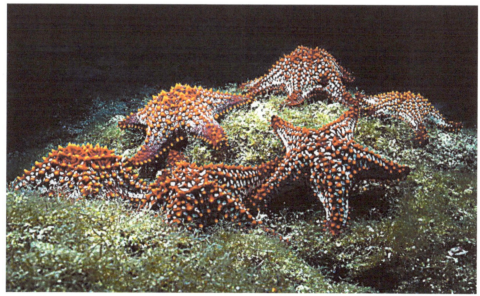

The big thick-armed cushion star is about 6 in. (15cm) across. They're found
mostly on the sandy bottom.

The **Middle Seamount** is probably the most abundant with life and also begins in the shallowest depth. There is one small area that begins at 50ft (15m), and then the rest of the plateau area is between 70-80ft (21-24m). At the edge of the plateau is a wall which drops to over 100ft (30+ m). The top of the mount is alive with clumps of coralline algae where hundreds of flower urchins live. At certain times of the year when the current picks up, they come out marching across the rocks releasing sperm and eggs in the current. Once this sex-march is over they rebury themselves in the algae. The middle seamount is also referred to as Moray Condos because of the great abundance of moray eels. In almost every crevice, a green head will be sticking out. The morays are found doubled and sometimes tripled up many with a large family all living in the same hole. An occasional green sea turtle, along with curtains of fish, surround the seamount's edges. Seen here often are schools of scissortail damselfish, king angelfish and barberfish. In the sandy patches what appears to resemble small craters is where triggerfish have laid their eggs. Many times, large groups of barberfish will have the little crater surrounded, swarming in to feed on the tasty morsels. Nearby, you'll usually see a frantic triggerfish darting back and forth in a defense mode.

In deeper water below 80+ ft (24+ m) while cruising the perimeter of the seamount, divers frequently see the schooling hammerhead sharks. They are found at different depths depending on the time of year, but usually in deep open water around pinnacles throughout the Sea of Cortez. Because of the surrounding upwelling, these prehistoric looking creatures feed on the pelagic fishes that also are part of this food chain. Other large fishes that are exciting to watch can be found over the seamount and around the deeper ledges, which include tuna, jacks and grouper.

Snorkeling over these seamounts can sometimes be very exciting offering great photo opportunities. Schools of pompano can be seen swimming just under the surface. Tiny 4 inch (10 cm) combed jelly fish drift through the water like some type of little alien as rainbow colors pulsate through their transparent bodies. They are beautiful to watch. But a few of the most exciting fishes that can occasionally be spotted while snorkeling here are the sleek billfish including marlin, sailfish and swordfish. The exquisite sailfish will open his iridescent blue-spotted sail when he spots you and then fold it down as he realizes that there is no danger. The billfish are very inquisitive and graceful, and it is a magical experience to meet one underwater.

## 33.  ISLA LAS ANIMAS

According to some local legend, spirits have been seen walking on Las Animas, which became known as the island of the spirits. There is certainly something spiritual about this island. It has phenomenal beauty both topside and underwater. There are three excellent dive spots: the island itself, the pinnacles and the seamount. Las Animas is an exciting colorful dive area.

**The Island (33A)  THE DEPTHS** around the island itself range from 20-100+ ft (6-30+ m). Divers can stay quite shallow and snorkelers can see a lot. But the slanting wall drops down to over 100ft (30m) quite rapidly. Sandy horizontal channels cut into the wall, leading divers to coral-covered overhangs, deep rock cavities and flat, sandy plateaus. Reef fishes and invertebrates are dense in the many crevices. There are usually a number of turtles on the reef structure surrounding the island.

On the northeast side of the island at 80ft (24m), there is a large opening to a cave which extends far back into the wall. The walls and ceiling of the cave are filled with golden cup corals and sometimes turtles are seen here catching a nap on the cave floor. Taking a dive light along to check out the walls of the cave opening is a good idea, as many fish and invertebrates display incredible colors.

**Caution:** No cave should ever be penetrated without proper training and equipment. At 60ft (18m) on the northwest side of the island is a shallower cave which does not extend back very far. This cave is interesting to check out as a variety of nocturnal creatures can be found, such as lobster, squirrelfish and shrimp.

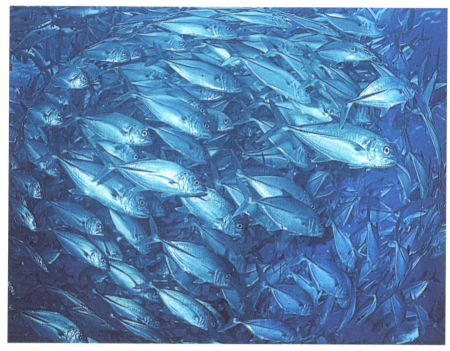

Found in schools of large numbers, during mating season, the male turns black, swimming beneath the female. After mating, he turns silver again.
"crevalle jacks"

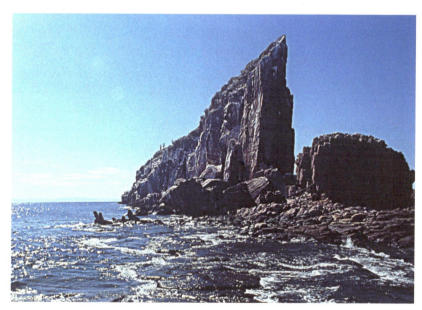

Isla Los Islotes sits offshore from La Paz and is home to a large sealion rookery.

## 34. THE PINNACLES

**THE DEPTHS** surrounding this site range from 40-120+ ft (12-36+ m). On the northwest side of the island are three pinnacles which protrude above the surface. The dive begins relatively shallow, then drops to great depths. On sunny days, rays penetrate between the massive boulders and jagged reef formations. Schools of small scissortail damselfish swim through these sun-dappled areas in swirls of thousands. The scissortail damselfish is characterized by its forked tail and white spot below the soft dorsal fin. They grow to only about 5 inches (13m), and are found in large numbers around reefs to depths of about 250ft (76m).

The walls of the pinnacles slope down in big sculptured steps to deep water. The steps form undercuts, ledges and a variety of small tunnels large enough for divers to swim through. The tunnels are fringed with purple and orange sea fans. A large variety of fishes are found around the entire perimeter. Some of them are the moorish idol and beautiful redtail triggerfish whose tail is lined with a brilliant blue border. The latter is also easily recognized by the blue streaks across its golden-colored head. Other fishes seen around the pinnacles are large grouper including the not so common golden grouper, leather bass, cabrilla and Pacific amberjack.

On the outer edges of the pinnacles, sometimes you can spot cruising hammerhead sharks as well as other large pelagics, such as tuna and several species of jacks. By swimming out a distance from the pinnacles at about a depth of 50-60ft (15-18m), divers commonly encounter massive schools of the big-eyed crevalle jacks. The average size of the jacks is about 50 lbs (23 kg) and they can be so thick that they are layered in the hundreds. At certain times of the year, they are seen in pairs swimming one atop the other. During this courting ritual the male will turn black and when the mating is over, become silver once again.

## 35. THE SEAMOUNT

**THE DEPTHS** here range from 45-130+ ft (14-39+ m) and this seamount is located off the south side of the island. The top of the seamount is at 45ft (14m) and has a relatively flat plateau covered with colorful sea fans and gorgonians. In between the coral fans are an array of reef fishes. Damselfish, rainbow and sunset wrasses, chromis, red longnose hawkfish and goby's fill the voids between the corals. Large schools of butterflyfishes and king angelfish seem more prevalent around the seamount than at many other sites. The walls of the seamount are quite steep and drop to depths of over 130ft (39m). Along these deeper ledges, divers can sometimes find hammerhead sharks at between 80-130ft (24-39m).

The seamount walls are lined with deep depressions. Tiny nudibranchs inch their way along the encrusting corals and sponges. Scorpionfish use coloring as protective camouflage. Since they lie still they are easy subjects for the photographer to frame. Many varieties of sea stars are also encountered here and include the chocolate chip, the orange star, the gulf star, the yellow-spotted star and the multi-armed crown of thorns.

The seamount is a fantastic spot with great photo opportunities. Just off the wall on the seaward side, large schools of crevalle jacks will usually linger. On this seaward side the currents can get extremely strong, so always beware. If the surface water is rippling over the top of the seamount like a little river, it's best to choose another dive spot.

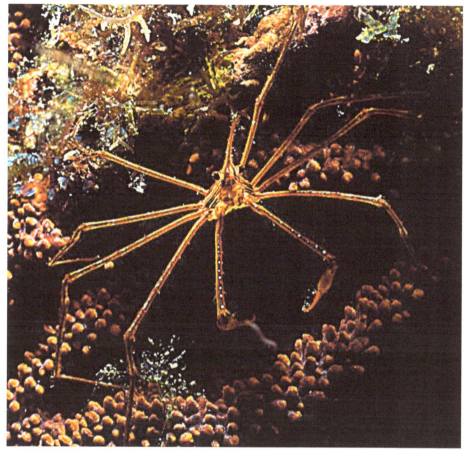

**The spider looking arrow crab is readily seen at night as it comes out to feed.**

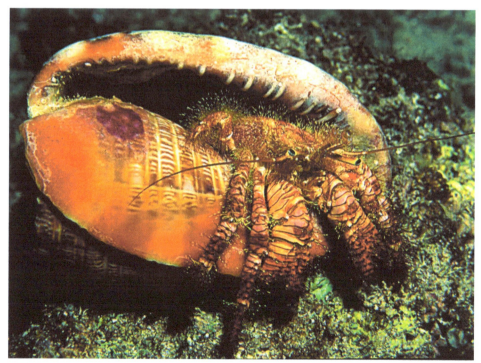

**The elegant hermit crab looks like a fuzzy little character. It's seen mostly at night when feeding.**

Just south beside the seamount which is out of the current run is the protruding **Sea Lion Rock**. Diving here starts in 5ft (1.5m) of water dropping to a 60ft (18m) sandy bottom. Sea lions frolic and play all around this rock, doing acrobatics for the cameras. Large schools of tropicals dart around the rock as if carrying on the sea lions acrobatic dance. This is also a great spot for snorkeling, as these playful water pups will float upside down a few feet beneath the divers, just observing the slow cumbersome humans.

## 36. ISLA SAN DIEGO

**THE DEPTH** ranges from 20-50ft (6-15m). Isla San Diego has a reef structure off its southwest side known as San Diego reef, which is a long, low-lying rock reef that breaks the surface. A diver can swim around the entire reef in one dive. On its south side is a labyrinth of caverns and grottos. These honeycombed passageways are great to explore as there is always some sunlight penetrating through the cracks and chimneys above. Cave-dwelling fishes that live in these darker waters have extremely large eyes. Sometimes a hundred or more squirrelfish, cardinalfish, soldierfish, glasseye and bigeye snappers are found bunched up together under the cavern ledges. Shimmering schools of thousands of tiny baitfish swirl around the entrance of the openings, forming a circle around divers as they enter. Cornetfish, trumpetfish and cortez angelfish are seen lingering close to the reef, darting in and out of the grottos doorways.

An uncommon fish in the Sea of Cortez is the leopard grouper, but it is frequently spotted solo at San Diego Reef. For some reason the ones here have turned golden and they are simply referred to as the golden grouper. Small schools of guinea puffers, chubs, grunts and surgeonfish are found clustered around the ends of the reef. Regularly seen around San Diego Reef are great schools of the Pacific crevalle jacks. Photographic opportunities are excellent in these schools as hundred of pairs of eyes, like polished mirrors, move straight toward the camera lens. The reefs outer walls are sprinkled with beautifully colored gorgonian corals which grow into the shape of oriental fans. The entire reef is nothing less than a three-tiered world of dramatic shapes and colors.

**Incredible Night Dive:** Night diving on this reef is equally incredible. The walls are a brilliant gold, covered with golden cup coral that open to feed on tiny planktonic animals drifting in the current. Anemones can be found in groups, transforming long vertical ledges into vibrant, living masterpieces. Nestled within the anemones are sleeping fish. Bright red shrimps, decorator crabs, arrow crabs and nudibranchs are milling about in search of food. Two interesting little critters are the decorator crab and the sponge crab. Both carry excess baggage on their backs. The decorator crab plants leafy algae on his entire body, while the little sponge crab places only pieces of sponge on his. (what's up with that?) At night, divers will often spot them when they notice pieces of algae and sponge moving slowly across the rocks.

The sandy bottom literally moves with the 3ft (1m) synapted cucumbers. Harmless but if touched, these cucumbers will stick to you like velcro. There is also a very unique worm called a nemertean (zebra) worm which only appears at night and has the coloring of a red-banded coral snake. Many divers mistake it for a snake. They are remarkably elastic and can stretch several times their body length, some to over 6ft (2m). They are predators and have a long proboscis which is thrust out to entangle prey such as small crustaceans and annelid worms, with paralyzing mucus.

Southeast of the exposed reef, at a depth of 60-75ft (18-23m) is a section of the reef seldom visited. When the current is flowing north, divers can venture out by panga for an excellent drift dive. If the current is flowing south, it is possible to dive a flat sandy area in 20-40ft (6-12m) of water that houses thousands of garden eels.

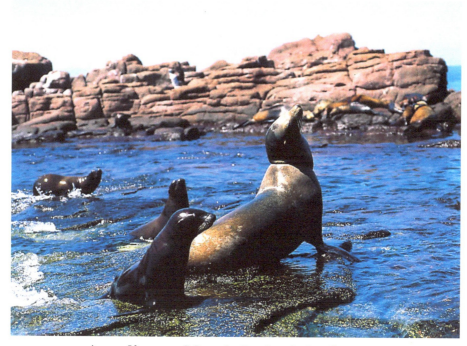

**A sealion and her baby bask in the sun.**

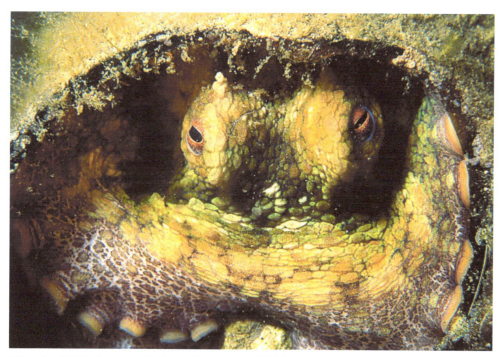

**Octopus like to hide in anything they can. This one just happens to be peeking out of a broken beer bottle.**

## 37. SALVATIERRA WRECK

**THE DEPTH** of this wreck is 60ft (18m). In 1975 the old La Paz to Topolobampo ferry, the 'Salvatierra', collided with some rocks and sank in the San Lorenzo Channel. The cargo consisted of trucks, many of which were salvaged, but remains are still scattered around. The props are still attached to the 300ft (91m) long hull which is still somewhat intact, and has been taken over by reef fish and invertebrate life. There are not many places to penetrate, but there are few openings in the wreckage to swim through. On a clear day this wreck is a great dive. Some of the largest known specimens of cortez angelfish have made this wreck their home. During the fall months, the beautiful iridescent blue and yellow striped juvenile cortez angelfish can be seen frolicking through the jumble. The wreck's skeletal cavities harbor green morays, jewel morays, frog fish and octopus, along with a variety of soft corals. Occasional schools of mobulas (a small-type manta ray) have also been sighted gliding over the wreckage. Cargo remains are strewn about the sandy bottom. Divers who look closely can find bullseye stingrays, round stingrays and halibut camouflaged between the debris.

**Caution:** Currents can really rip across the wreckage as it is not protected by any reefs. So, it is recommended to make your dives between these slack currents.

## 38. LA PAZ SHORELINE

**THE DEPTH** ranges from 6-30ft (2-9m) along La Paz's coastline. The coves in and around La Paz were once the center of much pirate activity. Construction on the main road in the 1970's gave credibility to the old pirate stories when a large chest of valuable silver and coins was discovered by workmen during the excavation. These coves are good spots for shore diving, but marine life is not nearly as abundant as that found around the offshore islands. There is some good snorkeling and shallow diving along the edges of the coves which reveal tropical fish life, along with invertebrates and mollusks. Easy entries are made as there is no surf. Drive 10 miles (16 km) north of La Paz and follow the main road to the ferry landing. Continue north along the waterfront and you will find the large **Bay of Pichilingue**. From here there will be another road that will continue on to Ballandra Bay which is also a large bay. There are several dirt roads which lead to coves. Any of the points off the coves can make for interesting underwater explorations.

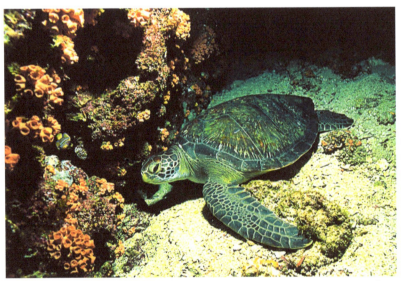

**The green sea turtle can be found around the reefs. They are often seen at night resting.**

# Chapter IX     EAST CAPE

*A Baja reality reminder... 'They laughed at Joan of Arc but she went right ahead and built it anyway'*

                                                                *(Gracie Allen)*

**About The Area:** Located halfway between La Paz and Cabo San Lucas, the East Cape area encompasses the southeast portion of the Baja peninsula. At one time this entire region was frequented by Spanish galleons and ravaging pirates. By the middle 1700's, virtually all the Indian population had died either of European diseases or in fighting with the Spanish. Surviving Indians were moved to the missions farther north, but the cape area and San Jose del Cabo remained an important Spanish military outpost until the mid-19th century when the presidio was turned over to Mexican nationals. Today, sailboats and private yachts can be found bobbing peacefully in the coves along the coastline. Miles of white sand beaches, rocky reefs and protected coves are only a short distance from the main roads.

**Getting There:** Alaska, Aeromexico, Aerocalifornia, Mexicana and American airlines all fly into Los Cabos. There are also airstrips for small private aircraft at several resorts. By vehicle, there is a turnoff from Highway 1 at Las Cuevas, which leads to the coastline and continues north to Punta Pescadero or south to San Jose del Cabo.

**Accommodations:** There are several resorts that offer excellent accommodations. The **Buena Vista Beach Resort**, the **Los Barriles Hotel** and the **Hotel Punta Pescadero.** A few other very nice resorts are the **Hotel Bahia Los Frailes,** the **Hotel Palmas de Cortez,** the **Rancho Leonero Resort** and **Hotel Playa del Sol.**

**Camping:** There are many beautiful white sand beaches along the coastline where you can set up a tent. For places that offer camping amenities, the **El Cardonal Resort** is a good choice. Also the **Punta Colorado** (from Buena Vista to Punta Colorado, a road runs a bit inland from the coast). There are stretches of open areas for beach camping here as well. Others are the **La Capilla RV Park,** the **Martin Verdugos Trailer Park** and **Los Cerritos RV Park.**

**Launch Ramps:** Larger boats can be launched at the **Martin Verdugos Trailer Park** at Los Barriles and at the **Playa de Oro RV Resort.** A few of the good hotels also have launch ramps. Inflatable and aluminum boats in the 12-15ft (3.6-4.5m) range are quite popular along the East Cape for beach launching.

**Diving Facilities:** There are a few diving operators from the East Cape area. Both **Pepe's Dive Center** and **Cabo Pulmo Divers** are located on the main road. Another shop is **Vista Sea Sports,** and **Cabo Pulmo Eco-Tours** is located in Costa Azul. Several of the hotels do offer diving services. They are the **Los Barriles Hotel,** the **Hotel Punta Pescadero,** the **Buena Vista Beach Resort** and **Rancho Leonero Resort.** And in Los Cabos there is **Baja Xplorer** at the Hotel Crown Plaza. They also give guided snorkeling tours.

**Diving and Snorkeling:** The entire Cabo Pulmo area is a protected marine park so the taking of all fish and shellfish is prohibited. Diving along the East Cape can be very exciting. To the south is Cabo Pulmo, where there is a hard coral reef. This coral ecosystem has created a beautiful natural aquarium. The rocky points which protrude from the peninsula offer an underwater terrain of large boulders creating a reef chiseled with narrow passageways and deep crevices. There is the remains of a wreck that lays strewn across the sandy floor, acting as a natural habitat for marine life. And there is Gorda Bank which lies further south. At certain times of the year Gorda Bank's deep water plateau attracts large pelagic fish including whale sharks and hammerhead sharks. The entire East Cape area, with its walls, ledges and reef systems, is teeming with a plethora of colorful marine life, which makes it a potentially rewarding area for photographers. Water visibility ranges from 60-100ft (18-30m) depending on the dive site. Clarity is better during the spring months. Water temperatures range from 65 degrees F (18C) in the early winter months to at least 80 degrees F (27C) in the late summer. The tides in this region are minimal compared to other northern areas in the Sea of Cortez. Rocky reefs which line the shore are excellent for snorkeling. Typical local reef fishes are in abundance as are a variety of shellfish, including the pink murex, spiny oysters, spotted cowries and pen scallops.

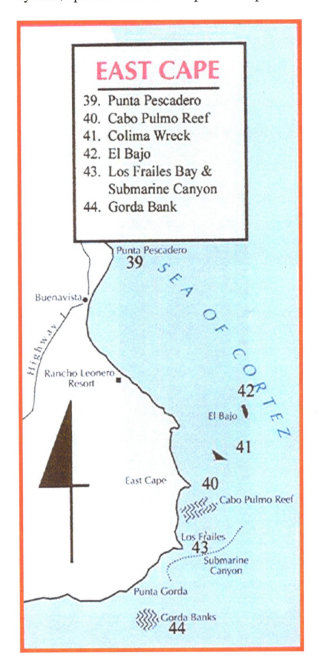

**EAST CAPE**
39. Punta Pescadero
40. Cabo Pulmo Reef
41. Colima Wreck
42. El Bajo
43. Los Frailes Bay & Submarine Canyon
44. Gorda Bank

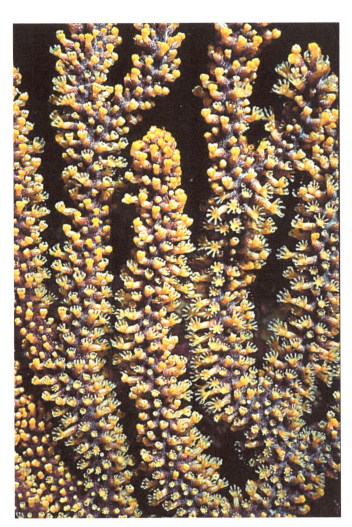

**Gorgonian corals are usually found along walls, where currents bring nutrients for them to filter feed.**

## 39.  PUNTA PESCADERO

THE DEPTH here ranges from approximately 25-80+ ft (6-24+ m). This point of Pescadero offers some great diving as well as good snorkeling. Large fish such as pargo, porgy, rock croaker, snapper and grouper can be encountered swimming over rocky boulders and through a catacomb of reef formations. The rocky bottom has a 20ft (6m) depth with a gradual slope which beckons divers to deeper water. Sandy channels cut through the reef like long fingers. Sitting almost motionless in the water, the Mexican barracuda with its sleek body and largemouth can sometimes be spotted hovering just over the sand as if on patrol. Also sitting practically motionless is the beautifully colored giant hawkfish which are easily camouflaged with their maze of wavy blue lines. Lizardfish, with their lizard-like bodies, are common here. They have the habit of resting high up on their pelvic fins.

Around the Pescadero point it is not uncommon to witness small schools of manta-like small mobulas swimming over the sand just beyond the rocks. There are literally hundreds of tropicals in this area, including barberfishes, triggerfishes, tangs and rainbow wrasse. Don't forget to look in the sandy patches, as sculpin, garden eels, stingrays and angel sharks inhabit this granular environment.

## 40.  CABO PULMO REEF

THE DEPTH ranges from 25-60ft (8-18m). The four finger-shaped reefs which stretch northeast from Pulmo Bay are known as Cabo Pulmo Reef. It is believed that this is the largest hard coral reef system on the western side of North America. Decorated with coral clusters in hues of green and gold, they are home to a myriad of reef dwelling animals and marine vegetation. Clusters of sea fans in shades of red and purple frame the narrow valleys and ledges. The reef is made up of short walls which drop from 25ft (8m) to 60ft (18m), where a sand bottom community dwells. Here are stingrays, snake eels and patches of hundreds of garden eels. Look for the gulf tulip snail, which is one of the largest reaching up to 1ft (30.5cm) in length. It is distinguished by its high spine and orange –brown shell. The reef has some large angular-shaped boulders that play teeter-totter over each other to form small grottos. The reef actually has the appearance of a fallen freeway overpass with chiseled channels zigzagging throughout. Almost every type of tropical fish can be found on Pulmo Reef. This natural setting has created an almost aquarium-like environment. Large game fishes are often seen among the outer reef areas, feeding on smaller fishes, while schools of brightly colored tropicals circumnavigate the entire area. The oddly-shaped body of the scrawled filefish, which is covered with blue-green scrawl marks and spots, are found among the coral clusters along with the black durgon, an uncommon triggerfish that can be found at times wedged into tiny rock crevices. Other triggerfishes, such as the blunthead and orangeside, are found in abundance. Also seen here are the large azure parrotfish with green bodies, each scale is outlined with orange and green streaks and brightly colored lines radiate from their eyes. There is usually a current running across the reef, so Cabo Pulmo is often a drift dive. Winds can pick up in the afternoon, causing waves to break against the shallower reefs, and creating uncomfortable surge and reducing visibility. But even on a bad day, visibility will usually average around 40ft (12m). Pulmo's beautiful montage of reef crests, ledges, deep crevices and drop-offs make this area outstanding.

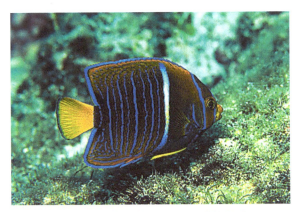

The juvenile king angelfish has iridescent colors of blue and gold stripes.

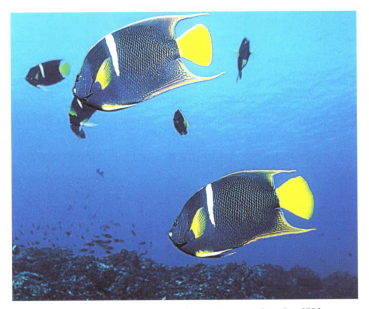

The adult king angelfish keeps its brilliant gold and blue but the colors begin to blend more.

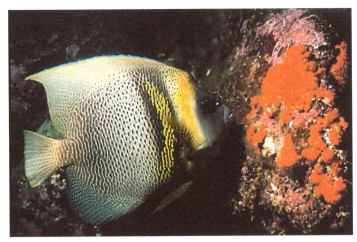

The gray and yellow cortez angelfish is found around the reefs throughout the Sea of Cortez.

## 41. COLIMA WRECK

**THE DEPTH** is around 40-50ft (12-15m). Located approximately 1 ½ miles (2.4 km) north of Pulmo Point lay the remains of the Colima, a large Mexican fishing vessel. The Colima hit the point during a storm in 1939 and was carried out to sea. It is now strewn across a sandy sea floor. Great masses of fishing net lie in clumps around the wreckage and entangled around the large prop. The rigging and sections of the torn hull harbor hundreds of fish. This wreck, now an artificial reef, should in fact be renamed 'pufferfish wreck', as so many pockets of the wreckage seems to be home to the slow moving glassy-eyed pufferfish.

Also schooling here is the elongated trumpetfish. In groups of about 20 or more, they hover over the great balls of fishing net. Schools of goatfish, each one ranging in the hundreds, linger over the wreck's skeletal remains along with grunts and snapper. Completely surrounding the main part of the dismembered hull are thousands of garden eels. They seem to be much larger and more approachable here than in other locations.

## 42. EL BAJO

**THE DEPTH** here is about 45ft (14m). The reef located just northeast of the Colima is known as El Bajo. Lying in the middle of a slow moving current, this reef is a maze of boulders and jagged rocky channels. Brilliant yellow porkfish can be found under ledges, bunched together in groups of dozens. Throughout the reef's long torso are many cortez and king angelfish, chubs, triggerfishes, parrotfishes and massive schools consisting of thousands of goatfish. Yellow, purple and red gorgonians cover the rocky terrain, forming an incredibly picturesque setting. This is another area where pufferfish are seen swimming in large groups. There are sandy channels that cut into the reef resembling man-made ditches. Above them are large overhangs that are covered with golden cup coral. Invertebrate life, such as the thick-spined pencil urchins, crown of thorns and sea stars, are grasping tightly inside the cracks. Shellfish are found clinging under overhangs. The beautiful pink-colored murex, spiny oysters, pen scallops and spotted cowries are just a few of the surprises that await divers. The visibility is usually 60-100ft (18-30m).

**Great Night Dive:** El Bajo also makes for a great night dive because the reef is covered with feeding golden cup coral. This area will invariably produce an incredible assortment of nocturnal creatures such as octopuses. Four kinds of lobster are residents of the reef; slipper lobster, blue spiny lobster, socorro lobster and the California spiny lobster. Brightly colored nudibranchs come out of hiding, along with basket stars, red shrimps and an array of crabs in all sizes and colors. Moray eels can be seen out of their holes hunting for food and on occasion several small opalescent squid are present.

## 43. LOS FRAILES BAY and SUBMARINE CANYON

**THE DEPTH** ranges from 15-100+ ft (5-30+ m). Still part of the protected marine park, Los Frailes Bay is reached either by boat or you can continue south about 2 miles (3.2 km) on the dirt road from Cabo Pulmo. The bay itself is protected from the prevailing northerly winds. Along the northern edge of Frailes Bay the rocky slopes follow down to the water and descend to shallow depths. The fallen boulders form a natural habitat for an abundance of marine critters. The sandy bottom reaches 60ft (18m) deep until it converges with a submarine canyon approximately a half mile (.8 km) out from shore. The steep canyon walls plunge to incredible depths. Their sheer sides are naturally carved with spectacular falls of cascading sand. For more advanced divers the shallower walls of the canyon are worth exploring. It is recommended to go with a local Divemaster that knows the area well. Divers have seen large grouper, black sea bass, jewfish, tuna, yellowtail, roosterfish, jacks, manta rays, turtles and an occasional lone shark along the canyon walls. Colorful sea fans line the vertical fissures which seem to go on forever.

## 44. GORDA BANK

**THE DEPTH** here begins at about 110ft (33m). Located 5 miles (8 km) off of Punta Gorda is an underwater seamount. The top of this huge mountain peak plateau is dotted with golden colored black coral bushes. In between these bushes are an abundance of moray eels. During certain times of the year, usually in the late fall, schooling hammerhead sharks are seen here. Depending on the seasons and currents, plenty of action is present in the first few feet of the water column. Whirlpools of jacks, Mexican barracuda, solitary manta rays, large tuna and on occasion sleek marlin have been sighted along with massive whale sharks. One never knows what they will or will not see but seamounts usually harbor a matrix of life forms. Due to the depth and unpredictable currents, this dive site is recommended for experienced divers only.

### HUMPBACK WHALES

Humpback whales first gained widespread public attention when scientists recorded their haunting songs. These complex melodies seem to be unique to each group of humpbacks, though they share certain common threads between groups. Just why they sing is not clear, although most of the vocalizing takes place in or near the mating grounds. Most of the humpbacks that spend the summer in the Gulf of Alaska migrate to Hawaii in winter. The whales seen in Baja are thought to be part of a population that spends the summer off the coast of central and northern California. The underside of their tail is like the fingerprints of humans, the pattern is different on each of them. In 1900, there were over 100,000 humpback whales. Commercial whaling has reduced that number to about 10,000. The females bear one calf every couple of years, so the humpback's comeback fight will be a long one.

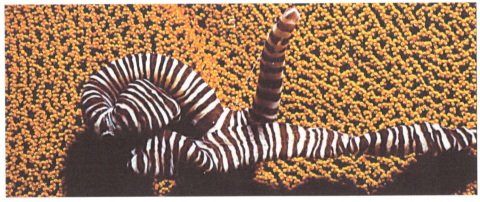

**The zebra worm resembles a sea snake and can stretch up to 12 ft (4m) in length. It hides in the daytime and can be found feeding on the reef at night. They prey on crustaceans using a paralyzing mucus.**

# Chapter X  CABO SAN LUCAS

A Baja reality reminder... 'Here is the test to find whether your mission on earth is finished; if you're alive, it isn't'
(Richard Bach)

## About The Area:

At the southernmost tip of Mexico's Baja Peninsula is the harbor at San Lucas, which English pirates were known to use as a hiding place from which to attack Manila galleons. Many of the historical incidents ascribed to Cabo San Lucas may actually have taken place near San Jose del Cabo, where ships often took on water from the Rio San Jose.

Today Cabo San Lucas is a tourist hot spot visited by thousands annually. Manila galleons have long since been replaced by private yachts, cruise lines and sport fishing boats. The area has good restaurants and hotels amidst an array of nightclubs, gift and craft shops. Outside of the busy hustle bustle town, Cabo's backdrop is rolling desert mountains and nice beaches with warm water in the summer and fall months. The main attractions include an underwater nature preserve and the naturally sculptured Land's End rock formations at one end of the bay. With the Pacific Ocean on Cabo's west side and the Sea of Cortez on its east side, Cabo's waters attract sun seekers and water sport enthusiasts of all kinds.

## Getting There:
Several major airlines fly into Los Cabos. They are Alaska airlines, America West airlines, Continental airlines, American airlines, Mexicana airlines and Aero California. If arriving by vehicle, Cabo San Lucas is the last stop on the peninsula off Highway 1.

## Accommodations:
Cabo San Lucas offers a wide variety of hotels and condos in all price ranges. The higher end hotels are the **Sheraton Hacienda del Mar**, the **Hotel Solmar**, the **Finisterra**, the **Hotel Hacienda Beach Resort**, the **Pueblo Bonito Rose**, the **Giggling Marlin Inn**, the **Aston Terrasol Cabo** and the **Plaza las Glorius**. The **Villa Stein** is a rental with a great view. A bit lower end hotels are the **Los Cabos Inn**, the **Medusa Suites**, the **Hotel Mar de Cortez**, and the **Hotel Dos Mares** among others.

## Camping:
There are quite a few places to set up camp. The **Club Cabo Motel and RV Campground**, which is ½ mile east of Club Cascadas, the **El Arco Trailer Park**, is 3.3 miles east of town on Highway 1, the **Vagabundos del Mar Trailer Park** is northeast of town off Highway 1, the **El Faro Viejo Trailer Park**, is in the northwest section of town, the **Paloma RV Village**, located behind the corona plant at the top of the hill, and the **Cabo Cielo RV Park**, that is northeast at Km 4 on the south side of Highway 1. There is a long, 33-mile stretch between **Punta Gaspareqo** and **Land's End** which is essentially one immense, unbroken beach. It's wide and backed by dunes, with soft white sand offering great opportunities for seclusion to those who are willing to hike. The slope is rather steep, and the surf pounds here, creating undertows that pose a serious threat to inexperienced swimmers. Still, surfers like riding the waves off the points on this coastline.

## Launch Ramps:
To reach the **Cabo Isla Marina ramp**, enter Cabo San Lucas on Highway 1 and go past the gas station half mile (.8 km) to the stop light. The ramp is to your left. It is 40ft (12m) wide, made of concrete and has good traction. There is also a **public ramp** which is 14ft (4.2m) wide, made of concrete and has good traction. When entering Cabo San Lucas on Highway 1, turn left one block past the stop light. Follow the road to the small traffic circle and turn left. The ramp is next to the Panga Hotel fleet.

**Diving Facilities:** There is **Blue Adventures, Andromeda Divers, Manta Divers, Dive Cabo San Lucas, Acuatica Los Cabos, Tio's Water Sports, Amigos del Mar** and in the Costa Real Cabo Resorts, there is **Lands End Divers, Neptune Divers, Underwater Diversions, Professional Diving Services** and **Deep Blue.**

**Diving and Snorkeling:** The Cabo San Lucas Bay is a protected underwater park and marine sanctuary. No marine life may be removed from the bay. The diving opportunities are varied and include suitable sites for all experience levels. Most of the diving is around the leeward side of the famous granite peninsula that divides the Sea of Cortez from the Pacific Ocean. A 1,000 ft (303m) submarine canyon lies 50 yards (45m) off the protected shoreline of the bay which creates a unique environment for large numbers of tropical fishes, invertebrates and plant life. The unusual sandfalls are one of Cabo's most popular dive sites.

Other classic dives off the cape are found at the end of the peninsula where the famous granite pillars and giant arch, both landmarks of Cabo San Lucas are located. The few scattered remains of a Japanese shipwreck lie just off Finisterra, meaning 'Land's End'. Most of the sites are protected from the wind and currents and the tides in this area are minimal. From June through October, there can be occasional heavy storms known as Chubascos. Water temperature generally ranges from high 60'sF (19-21C) in the early winter months to 85 degrees F (29C) in the late summer. Water visibility can exceed 100ft (30m). Territorial reef fishes common throughout the region include angelfish, butterflyfish, triggerfish, puffers, damselfish, moorish idols, parrotfish, perch and grouper. During the early spring months, the chances of seeing the California gray whale and the humpback whale are excellent but not guaranteed. Coming south from cold northern waters, the whales are in their calving and mating season.

Northeast of Cabo San Lucas on the way to San Jose del Cabo are a number of uncrowded, relatively pristine beaches, suitable for snorkeling, diving and camping.

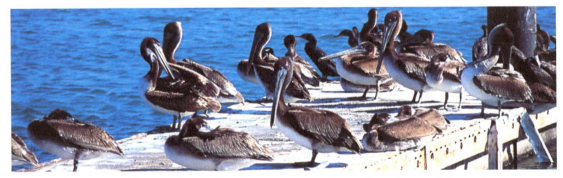

**Brown pelicans bask in the sun on piers, boats and beaches.**

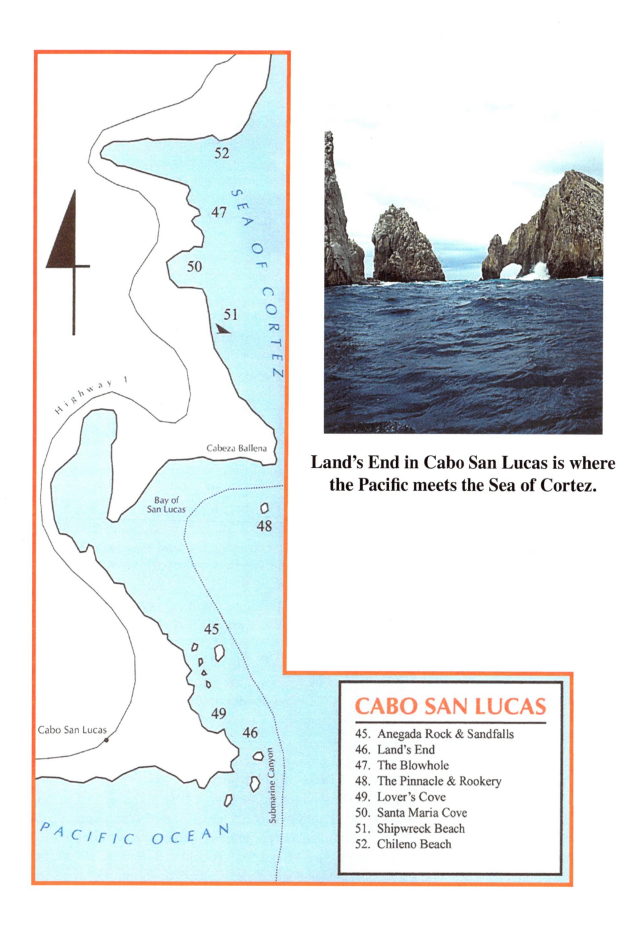

52

47

SEA OF CORTEZ

50

51

Highway 1

Cabeza Ballena

Bay of
San Lucas

48

45

49

Cabo San Lucas

46

Submarine Canyon

PACIFIC OCEAN

Land's End in Cabo San Lucas is where
the Pacific meets the Sea of Cortez.

## CABO SAN LUCAS

45. Anegada Rock & Sandfalls
46. Land's End
47. The Blowhole
48. The Pinnacle & Rookery
49. Lover's Cove
50. Santa Maria Cove
51. Shipwreck Beach
52. Chileno Beach

## 45. ANEGADA ROCK and the SANDFALLS

**THE DEPTH** ranges from 20-100+ ft (6-30+ m). **Anegada Rock** also known as Pelican Rock sits on the south side of the bay. On the sandy shallow bottom, schools of yellow barberfish, goatfish and king angelfish move back and forth on the shallower side of the rock. On bright days, flickering rays of sunlight bounce off this shallow sand area beside this great rock where reef fish seem to congregate. On these sunny days, the rock makes a beautiful backdrop for photos. By swimming south around the arch, divers will reach a year-round sea lion colony. The depth here is 40ft (12m).

Over the sandy 20ft (6m) ledge at Anegada Rock is a wall which drops down 1,000ft (303m) into a submarine canyon. Between depths of 50-100ft (15-30m), horizontal rocky outcroppings line the steep sloping wall, giving it the appearance of large jagged stair steps. The wall provides divers the opportunity to see an array of local tropical fishes and a chance encounter with manta rays, turtles and even possibly a whale.

At 90ft (27m) there is the **Sandfalls** made famous by Jacques Cousteau in a television documentary. At certain times of the year, large amounts of sand build up in shallower depths. When there is strong surge, the sand starts spilling down this sand valley resembling a giant white slide. It moves down the rocky wall to a depth of 100ft (30m) where the white granules meet a sheer granite wall. Here the sand drops straight down for hundreds of feet. The billions of falling granules resemble a waterfall in slow motion. It is an interesting dive especially from a geological perspective.

**Caution:** Because of the depth, the sandfalls should be dived by experienced divers.

## 46. LAND'S END

**THE DEPTH** here is 60ft (18m) and this is the location of Cabo's famous naturally-carved arch. Here at Land's End, years of wind and weather have hollowed out a beautiful archway through which the waves of the Pacific Ocean break meeting and merging with the waters of the Sea of Cortez. This dramatic topside setting extends beneath the water's surface into a beauty all its own. Giant angular rocks cascade down to a depth of 60ft (18m) where there is a sandy bottom. The short walls along the rocks are full of small ledges and indentations which create homes for large eels, reef fish and invertebrates. Beautiful moorish idols can be spotted swimming around in pairs, as can king angelfish and longnose butterflyfish. The rarely seen bright orange clarion angelfish is sometimes found at Land's End. This elegant-looking fish is normally a resident of the Clarion Islands and the Socorro Islands much further south.

There is sometimes a strong surge on the point at Land's End, but it is worth the swim as divers have had encounters with manta rays here. Other frequent visitors are sea turtles, large sea bass and schools of Mexican barracuda.

Several yards off the point's rocky outcropping is the partial skeletal remains of a Japanese fishing boat which met its doom in 1948. Today the wreckage is strewn across the sandy bottom in about 50ft (15m) of water. Fishes and invertebrates have made multi-condominium levels throughout the structures remains.

## 47. THE BLOWHOLE

**THE DEPTH** here ranges from 40-100+ ft (12-30+ m). This great rock sculpture gets its name from a blowhole in the rocks, where a small water surge is forced through a hole in the rock. The backside of this huge formation forms a wall which is filled with twisted crevices, rugged tunnels and deep ravines. Depths drop quickly to over 100ft (30m). Red and yellow gorgonians, along with sea fans, cover the area. Hard encrusting coral blankets the rocks in clumps. Frequently encountered in the shallower depths are hogfish, surgeonfish, croaker and porgies. Nurse sharks, sea turtles, jacks and guitarfish have been noted in this area along with a few large grouper.

## 48. THE PINNACLE and ROOKERY

**THE DEPTH** here is from 50-80ft (15-24m) and it is a good area to look for large fish. On occasion, divers have seen lone mantas swimming around the pinnacle. The pinnacle also harbors a community of sea lions which are always great fun to dive with. An entire dive can be spent just playing and photographing these jovial, fun-loving mammals. This area is alive with tropicals and invertebrate life. Look closely in the holes and rock fissures for the zebra moray. It is the only moray with white bands on a reddish brown body. Growing to a length of 4ft (150cm), these morays differ from others by having blunt, molar-like teeth instead of sharp canine teeth.

The bottom terrain levels off at a plateau around 50ft (15m), then slopes down to 80ft (24m). Currents have been known to pick up around the pinnacles, so the area is recommended for experienced divers.

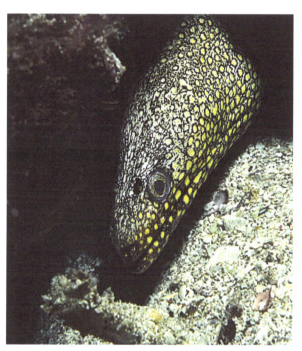

**With chainlike rows of gold rings on its body, the jewel moray can be found within the crevices of the reef.**

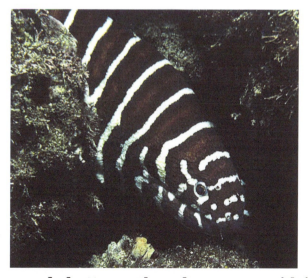

**Occasionally found on sandy bottoms, the zebra moray with its distinctive stripes, identifies it from others.**

## 49. LOVER'S COVE

THE DEPTH starts shallow at 10ft (3m), dropping to around 40ft (12m). Lover's Cove is located almost at the point of Land's End. It is most easily accessed by boat as water taxis shuttle between San Lucas and the cove every 20 minutes. To get there by foot, walk towards Land's End on the beach behind the Solmar Hotel. The cove does not have a lot to offer scuba divers, but there are some interesting rocks along the shoreline to snorkel around. There is one rock where several sea lions hang out, just basking in the sun and they are always a great joy to snorkel with.

## 50. SANTA MARIA COVE

THE DEPTH around this cove ranges from 15-60+ ft (5-18+ m). Located 7 miles (11 km) north of Cabo San Lucas, in front of the Twin Dolphin Hotel, is an excellent cove for shore diving as well as snorkeling. Parking is available in the hotel parking lot and there is a pathway on the left which leads to the mouth of the cove. The north point of Santa Maria Cove is made up of large rocks and finger ridges. Further out are deep canyons. The southern point of the cove is also fringed with large rocks and small caverns. Corals and sea fans are interspersed among the ridges, along with a kaleidoscope of tropical fish life. Small bright red coral hawkfish, longnose hawkfish, chameleon wrasses, sand perch, schooling spadefish, bluespotted jawfish and royal blue and yellow chromis are scattered in shallow water at 15-25ft (5-8m). Large game fish occasionally frequent the deeper areas by the tip of the points.

**Caution:** Currents can pick up around the points.

## 51. SHIPWRECK BEACH

THE DEPTH here is 30ft (9m). Just south of the Twin Dolphins Hotel which is 7 miles (11 km) north of Cabo San Lucas is Shipwreck Beach. In 1966 the Japanese freighter *Inari Maru* was wrecked on the shoreline. Part of the rusted hull lies on the shore, while the rest of the remains are scattered offshore in about 30ft (9m) of water. Easily reached from the beach, this is a good snorkeling and shallow scuba diving spot.

The Twin Dolphins Hotel is on the main highway. From the highway, turn at the Barco Varado sign which leads to the beach. Just beyond the beached remains of the wreckage, there is a series of long finger reefs. Being full of cubby holes and pockets, the rocky structure is home to an array of marine life. It is a good area for fish portraits if you are a photographer, as a variety of wrasses, blennies, trunkfish, rays and triggerfish live throughout the reef. Also some of the best snorkeling areas that can be reached from shore are from Shipwreck Beach to Santa Maria Cove.

## 52. CHILENO BEACH

THE DEPTH ranges from 10-50ft (3-15m). Located north of the Twin Dolphins Hotel which is 7 miles (11 km) north of Cabo San Lucas is Chileno Beach. It is located next to the Cabo San Lucas Hotel and is accessible by turning at the Cabo Real sign. Easy shore entries can be made in front of the hotel.

Protected finger reefs start right at the shore of Chileno Beach and jut out into the bay for about a half mile (.8 km). Divers will usually see a broad assortment of tropicals and eels, such as the striped zebra, tiger reef, tiger snake, jewel and green moray eel which hide in the deep fissures of the reef. Look towards the surface as many times the California needlefish swims inches below the surface in great schools. They have a slender elongated body with a knife-like snout. A wide variety of invertebrates stalk the outer fringes of the rocks, including the multi-petaled lavender flower urchin, brightly colored sea stars, hydroids and feather duster worms. This is also a very appealing area for snorkelers due to the shallower depths.

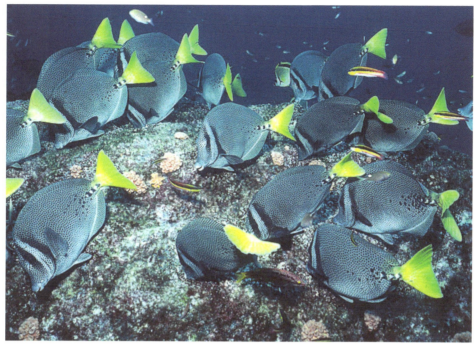

**About 2 ft (0.6m) in size, surgeonfish
are usually seen in schools around the reefs.**

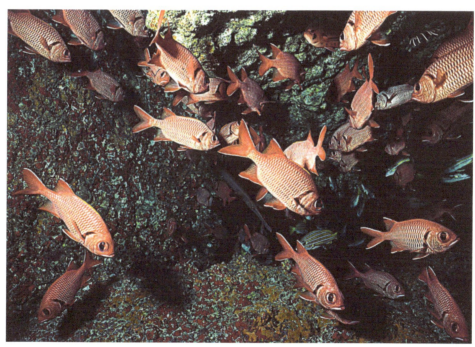

**The blackbar soldierfish, usually pinkish red in color is found under long, deep ledges
and in small caves and grottos.**

# Chapter XI  SOCORRO ISLANDS

*A Baja reality reminder... 'All truth passes through three stages. First, it is ridiculed; second, it is violently opposed; third, it is accepted as being self evident'*                                                                    (A.G., "Sculptor")

## About the Area:

Located 220 miles (355 km) south of Baja's tip sits a small group of volcanic islands, virtually in the middle of nowhere. The name of this island chain is Revillagigedo. There are four islands of which Isla San Benedicto is the closest to the Baja peninsula. Isla Socorro is 22 miles (36 km) further south, while Isla Roca Partida sits to the southwest. Isla Clarion is the furthest out in the Pacific, being 370 miles (597 km) from Baja's tip.

In 1952, Isla San Benedicto erupted, forming a prominent cone about 1,000 ft (303m) high, along with a large lava flow area which can be seen on its southern end. In January 1993, Isla Socorro awoke from 145 years of dormancy when a fissure opened on the ocean floor, spewing huge rocks as large as 10ft (3m) in diameter. These rocks were filled with gas and floated on the surface until the gas dissipated. Except for a small Mexican naval base which is there to enforce regulations and a village on the southern tip of Isla Socorro, the islands are uninhabited. This archipelago has been referred to as the Mexican Galapagos. The birds seem fearless and many are endemic to the area, as are several plants. A story by one biologist who was doing research was that when he was napping, a Socorro wren landed on his belly, hopped up to his chest, and looked intently at the folds in his shirt and even up his nose for morsels to eat. So lack of fear by human intrusion was yet unknown. This is one of the only places that we have witnessed sharks and dolphins interacting. At night when the boat was at anchor, hundreds of flying fish were jumping from the water, attracted to the boats lights. Dolphins and galapagos sharks were nose to nose bumping each other in competition for this tasty feast. There did seem to be a certain respect paid to the dolphins from the sharks though. But complete harmony and respect seemed to exist between both.

Almost every hurricane that originates in the Pacific and heads for Mexico and Central America moves through this archipelago. Because of the unpredictable weather, these islands are only visited by long-range boats and commercial tuna vessels. All boats traveling to these islands need special permits from the Mexican government. The hurricane months are from June to October, with occasional storms in May and November. During the winter months from late October through May, the weather conditions can, at times, exhibit strong winds and heavy seas. The most stable weather conditions are in November to early December and in April and May. In the fall, the water temperature is around 80 degrees F (27C), while in the spring it is about 70 degrees F (21C).

A presidential decree in 1994 declared the Socorro Island chain a national protected biosphere reserve. No collecting or fishing is allowed within 12 miles of the inland waters. There has been much controversy over the commercial fishing here. After a dive boat videotaped the incredibly sad and gruesome slaughter of many of the friendly giant manta rays at 'the Boilers' in February of 1994, a public outcry and demand to protect the Socorro islands grew. But this area as well as the entire Sea of Cortez is still in much need of adequate patrolling and law enforcement to protect its most valuable asset, which is the incredible marine life that thrives beneath its waters.

## Getting There: 
The best way to get to the Socorro Island chain is by boat. There is a small airstrip on Socorro, but it is not commonly used. Departing from Baja's tip at Cabo San Lucas, most dive boats take approximately 24 hours to arrive at Isla Benedicto. A few dive boats do come out here on a regular basis. One is the Solmar V, a 112ft (34m) liveaboard boat with 12 cabins. Another is the Fiesta, a large liveaboard which offers longer excursions. Both are based out of Cabo San Lucas.

**Diving and Snorkeling:** Diving at the Revillagigedo Islands is a unique experience. Due to their isolation from the mainland, these islands are home to a variety of endemic plant and animal species. Below the surface of the surrounding Pacific Ocean, the islands are renowned for their prolific marine life, including giant manta rays, many shark species, large pelagic fish such as marlin, yellowfin tuna, jacks, wahoo, dolphins and whale sharks. You can expect to see large schools of the brightly orange colored clarion angelfish and the elegant redtail triggerfish. In the spring months, divers have a good chance to see humpback whales. Being of volcanic origin and because of the swift hurricanes that move through this area, the topside is quite barren. Likewise, the underwater terrain is void of gorgonians and soft corals. Consisting of grey rock formations with only a small amount of hard coral, the scenery is generally unattractive but it is offset by large marine animals and clear blue water. The most visited islands for divers are Isla San Benedicto, Isla Socorro and Roca Partida. The islands do offer some good snorkeling. Shallow reefs and sites such as the Boilers on Isla San Benedicto, are great for snorkeling. Snorkelers can interact with the giant mantas as they frequently hang around on the surface. Other islands where there is a lot of shark activity, snorkeling can be exciting, but tank diving is recommended.

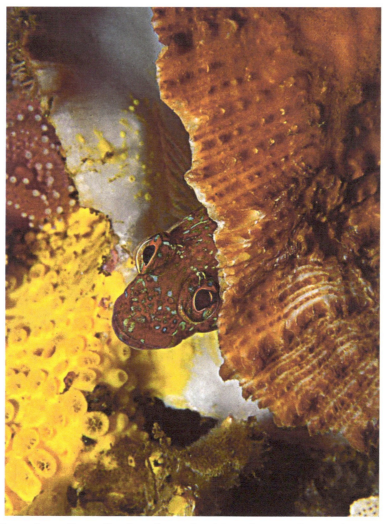
**Blennies often find refuge inside of a variety of shells.**

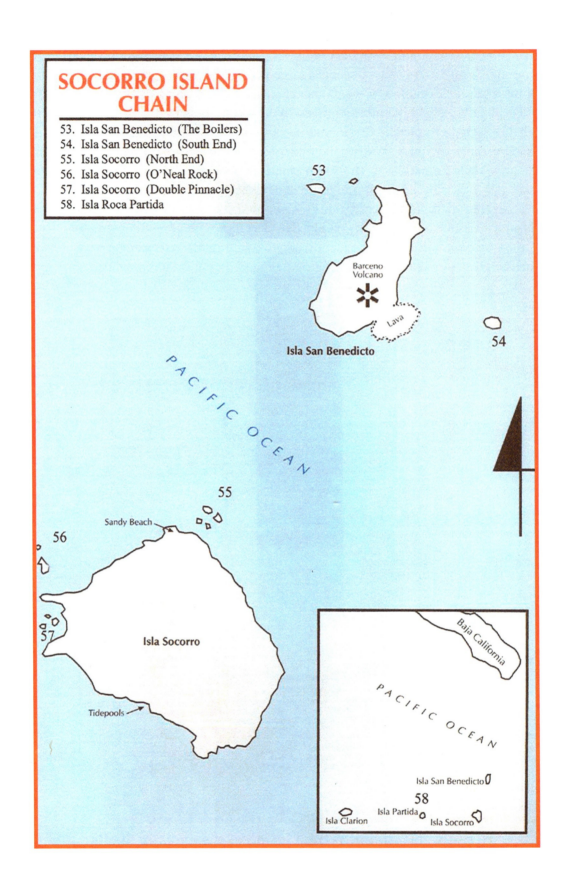

# SOCORRO ISLAND CHAIN

53. Isla San Benedicto  (The Boilers)
54. Isla San Benedicto  (South End)
55. Isla Socorro  (North End)
56. Isla Socorro  (O'Neal Rock)
57. Isla Socorro  (Double Pinnacle)
58. Isla Roca Partida

53

Barceno
Volcano

Lava

54

**Isla San Benedicto**

PACIFIC OCEAN

55

Sandy Beach

56

57

**Isla Socorro**

Tidepools

Baja California

PACIFIC OCEAN

Isla San Benedicto

58

Isla Partida

Isla Clarion

Isla Socorro

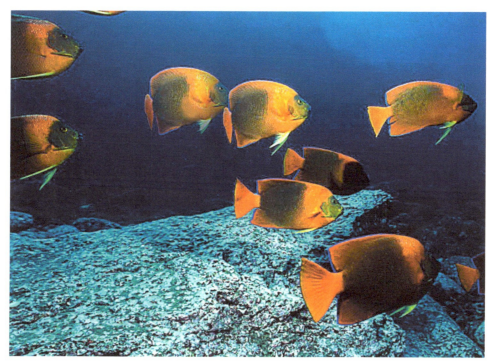

The clarion angelfish is a beautiful orange. They are sometimes seen in the southern part of the Sea of Cortez, but mainly further south in the Islas Revillagigedo. They clean parasites off of manta rays.

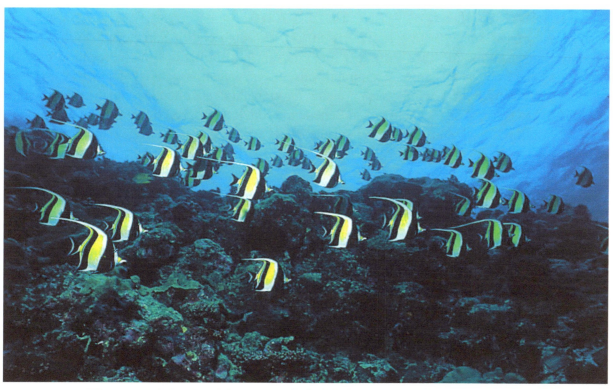

The exquisite looking moorish idols are rarely seen alone.
They swim in pairs or more.

## 53. ISLA SAN BENEDICTO    The Boilers

**THE DEPTH** ranges from 25-100+ ft (8-30+ m). One of the most picturesque dive sites at Isla San Benedicto is known as 'The Boilers', located at the northwest end. It is an underwater pinnacle that starts in 25ft (8m) of water. This shallow plateau extends approximately 100ft (30m) across. The sides of the pinnacle are vertical walls that drop to a 120ft (36m) sandy bottom. The top of the pinnacle is absolutely alive with color as are its side walls. The exotic-looking black and gold moorish idols, usually seen in pairs can be found here in schools of great numbers. Neon orange clarion angelfish, pufferfish, wrasses, hogfish and redtail triggers are also abundant. Whale sharks have been known to linger around the pinnacle during both fall and spring months.

But the main attraction of this seamount is the likelihood of seeing the giant manta rays. With 18+ ft (5+ m) wing spans and a weight of up to 3100 pounds, these exquisite friendly creatures seem to be as curious about divers as the divers are about them. They are gigantic filter-feeders, straining the water for plankton and small fishes through their very wide, rectangular mouths. Lobes on the sides of their heads are unfurled when the animals are feeding, funneling water and food into their massive mouths. Being one of the most docile animals in the sea, these eminent beauties seem to really enjoy human contact. After spending a good amount of time with these creatures, it is easy to see why studies are beginning to show their intelligence. It is suspected that they will soon be high on the list of respected animals, as are the dolphins and whales.

Around the seamount are columns of silver swirls, which consist of hundreds of both amberjacks and horse-eyed jacks. Occasionally solo tuna and wahoo will dart by. Beyond the seamount in deeper water, divers can sometimes spot hammerhead sharks. A little closer to the island, approximately 75 yards (68m) from the shore is another seamount that comes to within 80ft (24m) of the surface. It is a good spot to find larger fish weaving their way across the reef top.

## 54. ISLA SAN BENEDICTO    South End

**THE DEPTH** ranges from 40-100+ ft (12-30+ m). At the south end of San Benedicto there appears to be more shark activity. At 40ft (12m), this rocky terrain has formations that descend to over 100ft (30m). Sharks that frequent this area are hammerheads, silkys, whitetips, galapagos and gray reef sharks. Occasionally a lone tiger shark will be seen cruising through. At deeper depths schooling hammerheads are more likely to be seen. Sharks here at San Benedicto seem less spooked by divers and are fairly easy to approach. Both the south end and east side of the island are great sites for diving and are still a shark photographer's paradise.

## 55. ISLA SOCORRO    North End

**THE DEPTH** ranges from 30-100+ ft (9-30+ m). The island of Socorro is larger than San Benedicto. On the northeast side of the island divers can sometimes find a fair amount of shark activity. The area can get some pretty strong currents, so drift diving is often the choice. At the north end, there are some protruding rocks that jut out from the island. Underwater at about 50ft (15m) and deeper, the terrain is made up of large, flat and oblong boulders. Here, there are great schools of clarion angelfish and redtail triggerfish. As you ascend to about 30ft (9m), the terrain takes on a whole new appearance. The incredible volcanic earth formations look like something you might expect to see on the moon. There are great angular channels in the reef to swim through which are dotted with pockets. These pockets make perfect homes for eels, octopus, urchins, starfish and large socorro lobster.

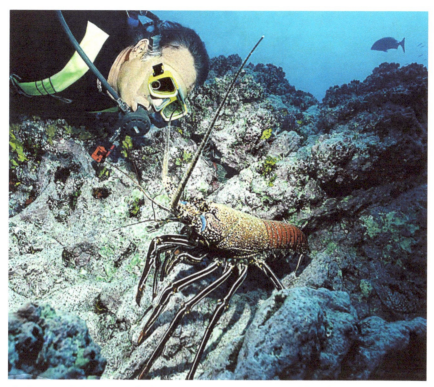

A large Socorro lobster comes out to check out a diver.

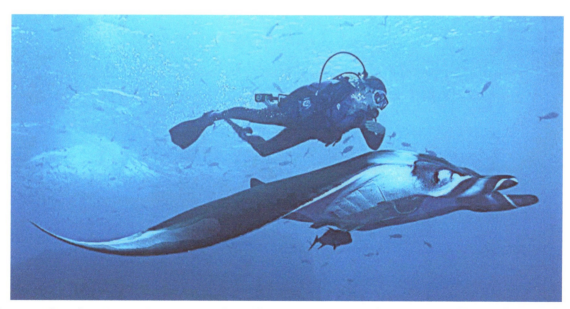

The gentle giant manta rays enjoy diver contact and are as curious about divers as we are about them.

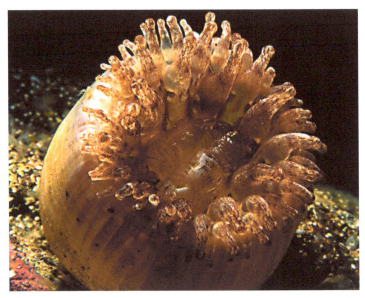

**Sea anemone's of all shapes and colors are found throughout the reefs and on the sandy bottom.**

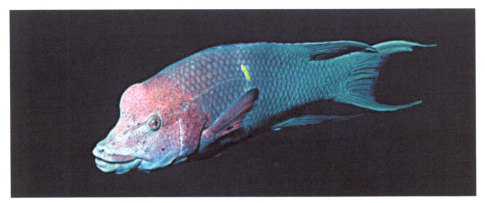

**Mexican hogfish are similar to the California sheepshead.**

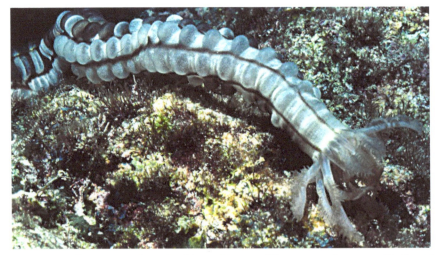

**At night, the synapted cucumber is found crawling on the sandy bottom. They are up to 50 in. (120cm) in size, and when touched they will stick to you like velcro.**

## 56.  ISLA SOCORRO    O'Neal Rock

THE DEPTH here ranges from 40-100+ ft (12-30+ m). This site on the northwest side of the island has several different names depending on the dive boat you're on, but the most common are O'Neal Rock and Old Man Rock. There is a large rocky plateau at 40ft (12m) where big lobsters, rays and a myriad of fishes can be found. Scorpion fish and octopus become camouflaged in the rocks and large eels poke their heads out from crevasses. On the outer edge of the plateau is a drop-off. Below the drop-off on the wall at 90ft (27m), there is a cavern with a large arch above it, which is a dramatic backdrop for photographers. Along the wall is a good area to look for schooling hammerhead sharks. Sometimes they will be seen in pairs or small groups swimming gracefully over the shallower plateau.

## 57.  ISLA SOCORRO    Double Pinnacle

THE DEPTH ranges from 30-100+ ft (9-30+ m). On the west side of the island high above the water's surface, there is a double set of rocks which resemble a manta ray's horns. Named the Double Pinnacle, or sometimes called Manta Rock, the great boulders that make up this reef formation lie between 30-50ft (9-15 m) in depth. The crevices lined between the boulders are great places to find large moray eels and lobsters. There also seem to be many juvenile whitetip sharks in this area. At a 50ft (15m) depth, the boulder covered plateau plunges to over 100ft (30m). Along this wall there is an array of fish life, including trumpetfish, triggerfish, large jacks and schools of chubs. Located on the southwest side is the **Tidepools** or **Aquarium** which is a large pool that inhabits juvenile fish and invertebrates. This is a great area for both diving and snorkeling.

## 58.  ISLA ROCA PARTIDA

THE DEPTHS here start shallow right against the sheer rock walls of this island and drop down into the big blue yonder. Roca Partida is the smallest and most isolated of the Revillagigedo islands. It rises from the deep blue and is a magnet for big marine life. It is a guano covered white rock that is small enough that a diver can easily swim around it during a single dive. The main thrill here is all the sharks. Whitetips, Galapagos and hammerheads are seen regularly. Some manta rays and occasional whale sharks cruise through this area. The underwater walls on this island are sheer and most of the dive is done in blue water, keeping the island walls in sight as a reference point. Beneath you, there are usually cruising sharks deep down in the blue. This is one of the most exciting dives as you never know what you will see. Large pelagic fish are the norm and visibility is usually over 100ft (30m). If you want big and wild, this is the place to go.

A Baja reality reminder... 'AND ALWAYS REMEMBER:  Humpty Dumpty was pushed!'

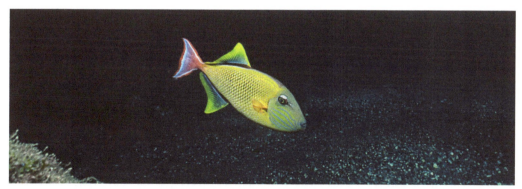

**The redtail triggerfish will sometimes be seen in the southern part of the Sea of Cortez, but larger schools are found in the Islas Revillagigedo.**

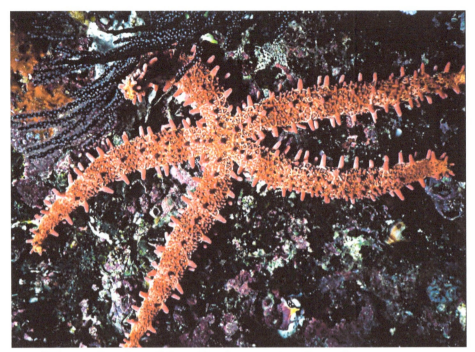

**The red colored bradley's sea star is quite common.**

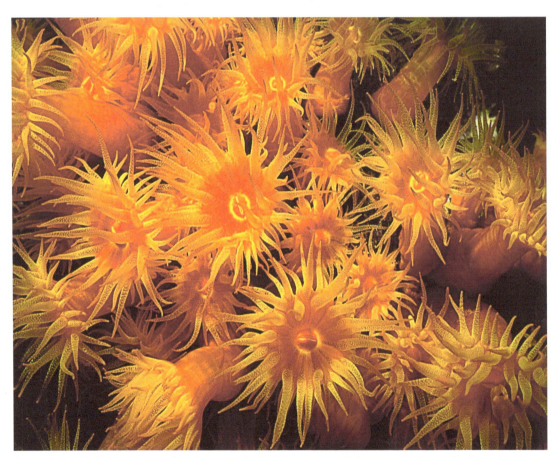

**Golden colonial cup coral open and feed under ledges and at night. Some walls will be blanketed with them.**

# Appendix

## Scuba Diving Centers

**Note:** Calling Baja from the U.S. or Canada, dial 011 for international access, then the country code which is 52 + area code + number.

## Bahia De Los Angeles

**Camp Gecko**
Email: gecko@starband.net

**Daggett's Campground**
Email: Rubendaggett@hotmail.com

**Archelon**
Email: resendizshidalgo@yahoo.com

**Raquel's**
Email: bahiatours@yahoo.com

## Mulege

**Cortez Explorers**
Moctezuma 75-A
Mulege BCS 23900
Email: info@cortez-explorer.com
www.cortez-explorer.com

## Loreto

**Dolphin Dive Center**
Ave. Benito Juarez
e/ Calle Davis y Lopez Mateos
Loreto BCS 23880
Ph: 613-13-51914
Email: dolphindivebaja@yahoo.com
www.dolphindivebaja.com

**Las Parras Tours**
Fco. I. Madero #16
Loreto BCS
Ph: 613-13-51010
Email: lasparras@prodigy.net.mx
www.lasparrastours.com

**Danzante Resort**
PO Box 94
Loreto BCS 23880
Ph: 613-10-40607
Email: info@danzante.com
www.danzante.com

**Baja Outpost**
Adolfo Lopez Mateos
Loreto BCS
Ph: 613-13-51134
Email:outpost@bajaoutpost.com
www.bajaoutpost.com

**Cormorant Dive Center**
Fco. 1 Madero
Loreto BCS
Ph: 613-104-2468
Email: cobadi@hotmail.com
www.loretours.com

**Empresas Rojo** – marine equipment
Calle Davis y Juarez
Loreto BCS
Ph: 613-13-50807
Cell: 612-12-71518

## La Paz

**Baja Quest**
Rangel #10 e/Sinaloa y Sonora
La Paz BCS 23060
Ph: 612-12-35320
Email: bajaquest@prodigy.net.mx
www.bajaquest.com.mx

**Baja Expeditions**
2625 Garnet Ave
San Diego, CA 92109
Ph: 800-843-6967
Email: travel@bajaex.com
www.bajaex.com

**Baja Diving & Service/Club Cantamar**
A. Obregon 1665-2 Plaza Cerralvo Ctr.
La Paz BCS
Ph: 612-12-27010
Email: info@clubcantamar.com
www.clubcantamar.com

**Scuba Baja Joe**
APDO Postal 588
La Paz BCS CP 23000
Ph: 612-12-40001
530-953-7567  U.S.
Email: bajajoe@yahoo.com
www.bajajoe.com

**Cortez Club**
La Concha Hotel
Km 5 Carr. Pichilingue
La Paz BCS
Ph: 612-12-16120
Email: info@cortezclub.com
www.cortezclub.com

**Carey Outdoors**
3956 Texas St. #16
San Diego, CA 92104
Ph: 619-701-6868/ 888-265-4141 U.S.
Email: reserve@carey.com.mx
www.carey.com.mx

**Sea & Adventures**
564 Topete Interior
E/5 de Febrero y Navarro
La Paz BCS
Ph: 612-12-30559/ 800-355-7140 U.S.
Email: mya@kayakbaja.com
www.kayakbaja.com/scuba.html

**Tio's Sports**
(located in front of Melia Hotel)

**Fun Baja**
Km 2.5 Carretera a Pichilingue
Marina Palmira, suite 15
La Paz BCS
Ph: 612-12-52366
Email: infogrupo@funbaja.com

# East Cape

**Pepe's Dive Center**
PO Box 532
Cabo San Lucas BCS 23410
Ph: 614-14-10001

**Cabo Pulmo Divers**
(located on main road)
Ph: 624-13-00235

**Vista Sea Sports**
Apartado Postal 42
Buena Vista BCS 23580
Ph: 614-14-10031
Email: vseasport@aol.com

**Cabo Pulmo Eco Tours**
(located in Costa Azul)
Ph: 614-14-45353

**Cabo Pulmo Dive Center**
Cabo Pulmo Beach Resort
Ph: 624-14-10244

# Los Cabos

**Baja Xplorer** (Hotel Crown Plaza)
Ph: 624-14-29292 ext. 714
Email: service@bajaxplorer.com
www.bajaxplorer.com

# Cabo San Lucas

**Blue Adventures**
At Fiesta Marina Hotel
Ave. Azul S.A. de C.V. Marina Cabo Plaza
Local 39K Cabo San Lucas BCS 23410
Ph: 624-14-44680/ 602-324-9007 U.S.
Email: blueadventuresdiving@yahoo.com
www.aventurasazul.com

**Andromeda Divers**
(next to office & Billygans Restaurant)
Playa Medano Beach
Ph: 624-14-32765
Email: m31dive@prodigy.net.mx
www.scubadivecabo.com

**Manta Divers**
Paseo del Pescador #1, Playa Medano
Cabo San Lucas BCS
Ph: 624-14-43871
Email: mantacabo@yahoo.com

**Dive Cabo San Lucas**
Email: info@cabovillas.com
www.divecabosanlucas.com

**Acuatica Los Cabos**
(in the Hilton Hotel)
Ph: 624-14-77084

**Tio's Water Sports**
(located on Melia Beach)
Ph: 624-14-32986
Cell: 624-11-81272

**Amigos del Mar**
PO Box 43, Cabo San Lucas BCS
Ph: 624-14-30505
Email: caboresort@aol.com
www.amigosdelmar.com

*Note: The following Dive Operators are located in the 'Costa Real Cabo Resorts' formerly the 'Plaza las Glorius'*

**Land's End Divers**
(Costa Real Cabo Resort)
Cabo San Lucas BCS
Ph: 624-14-32200
Email: landsenddivers@prodigy.net.mx

**Neptune Divers**
(Costa Real Cabo Resort) Local A-18
Cabo San Lucas BCS
Ph: 624-14-37111
Email: neptunedivers@cabotel.com.mx

**Underwater Diversions**
(Costa Real Cabo Resort)
Loc. #F5,6,7 Blvd. Marina
Cabo San Lucas BCS
Ph: 624-14-34004
Email: diversions@prodigy.net.mx
www.divecabo.com

**Professional Diving Services**
(Costa Real Cabo Resort)
Cabo San Lucas BCS
Ph: 624-14-31070

**Deep Blue**
(Costa Real Cabo Resort)
Cabo San Lucas BCS
Ph: 624-14-37668

# Islas de Revillagigedo (Socorro Is.)
**Solmar V**
PO Box 383
Pacific Palisades CA 90272
Ph: 800-344-3349
Email: caboresort@aol.com

**Fiesta**
(Reservations) call Fernando Aguilar
Ph: 612-122-1826
    612-122-7010
Email: info@clubcantamar.com
www.clubcantamar.com

# Index

# About the Authors

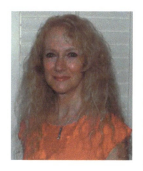

**SUSAN SPECK** is a Divemaster and currently co-owner of Dolphin Dive Center in Loreto Baja. She has owned and managed a dive store in California for 24 years and has been photographing and diving the Sea of Cortez for more than 25 years. Her articles and photographs of Baja and many other remote diving destinations have appeared in diving, travel and nature magazines worldwide. She also authored the book 'Diving Baja California', by Aqua Quest Publications in 1995. She served on the Board of Directors for CEMR 'Coalition for Enhanced Marine Resources'. Having studied marine life sciences, she has a special fondness for the Sea of Cortez. She has traveled extensively throughout the world, and has been one of first to dive many primitive and remote areas. She was on the first dive expedition to Sipadan Island in Malaysia, camping in tents. She continues to lead dive expeditions worldwide.

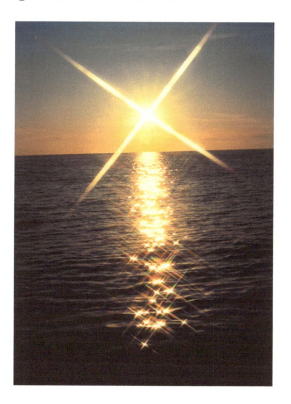

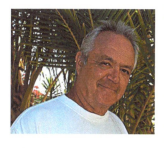

**BRUCE WILLIAMS** is a Master Scuba Instructor and has a degree from Pepperdine University, CA. He is currently co-owner of Dolphin Dive Center in Loreto. He owned and operated a dive store in California for 10 years. His photography has appeared in dive publications and calendars. He also gives presentations on diving and marine life from his extensive expeditions worldwide. He began exploring Baja in 1964, driving the entire peninsula in a fiat when the roads were unpaved. With his great passion for Baja, through his talks and photography, he strives to show others the richness of the Sea of Cortez.

CPSIA information can be obtained
at www.ICGtesting.com
Printed in the USA
LVHW071506260123
738003LV00002B/39